P L A N E T
C A N C E R

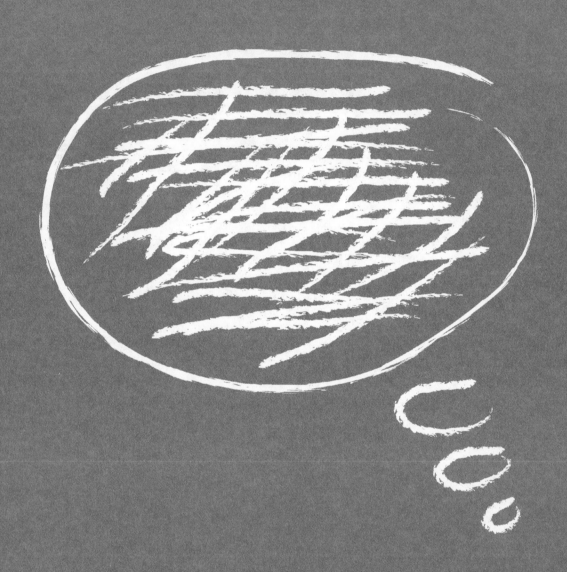

PLANET CANCER

The Frequently Bizarre Yet Always Informative
Experiences and Thoughts of Your Fellow Natives

Heidi Schultz Adams **and** Christopher Schultz

LYONS PRESS
Guilford, Connecticut

An imprint of Globe Pequot Press

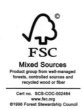

To buy books in quantity for corporate use
or incentives, call **(800) 962-0973**
or e-mail **premiums@GlobePequot.com.**

Lyons Press is an imprint of Globe Pequot Press.

Illustrations © Nadyne Wood

Text design by Sheryl P. Kober

Library of Congress Cataloging-in-Publication Data
Adams, Heidi Schultz.
  Planet cancer : the frequently bizarre yet always informative
experiences and thoughts of your fellow natives / Heidi Schultz Adams
and Christopher Schultz.
    p. cm.
  ISBN 978-0-7627-5901-9
  1. Cancer—Popular works. 2. Cancer—Computer network resources. 3.
Cancer—Patients—Services for. I. Schultz, Christopher. II. Title.
  RC263.A32 2010
  616.99'400285—dc22

                                                    2010023105

Printed in the United States of America

10 9 8 7 6 5 4 3 2 1

Planet Cancer: People Who Get It

Planet Cancer? WTF? You or someone you know has landed here, and it feels pretty solitary. Probably all you see in the waiting rooms are patients who are either much younger or much older than you—as you flip through either Highlights or the AARP magazine. But believe it or not, plenty of people your age have cancer—more than you think. In fact, nearly seventy thousand young adults (ages fifteen to thirty-nine) are diagnosed each year with cancer in the United States.

So . . . where the hell are they?

They're in no-man's-land. Young adults with cancer have fallen through the cracks in our medical system, which has a hard divide between the pediatric and adult cancer worlds. Children under fifteen and adults over forty are well-served cancer communities with plenty of dedicated resources, research, and targeted support. No such attention has ever been paid to young adults. As a result, cancer is the leading cause of death due to disease in young adults, and survival rates for this age group haven't improved in thirty years.

When Heidi was diagnosed at age twenty-six, she only met four other young people close to her age during eighteen months of treatment and its aftermath. They got close, and fast. Although they didn't know much about each other's "real" lives, they bonded in that place where they had been exiled with a single diagnosis: the place they named Planet Cancer.

On Planet Cancer, nothing was off-limits. They dove right in and talked about all the things that they could only discuss with each other. Things that caused nervous eye rolls in family members and well friends: vomit and constipation, mouth sores, living and dying, and whether one could be buried in blue jeans. Not only did they talk about these things, they actually laughed about these things. And in that laughter was born a deep friendship.

Three of the four friends died within the year they met. But out of that initial friendship, Planet Cancer was born as a place for young adults to find each other, to connect, and to forge the same bonds that Heidi and John and Robin and Paul had created.

First came a Web site and some message boards; now Planet Cancer serves young adults all over the world who populate its virtual community and attend its in-person retreats. They communicate, they educate, they support each other, encourage each other, scold each other and, perhaps just as important, they laugh together. In 2009 Planet Cancer joined forces with Lance Armstrong Foundation, turbocharging the mission and bringing young adult voices to the table to address other pieces of the problem, like the lack of research on young adult cancer and the gap in medical professional education.

See, we hate cancer. But we believe that the cancer experience can be transformed when you are able to share it—the good, the bad, and the very, very ugly—with someone else who "gets it" by virtue of having been there too. When you become part of a community like Planet Cancer, where everyone is facing the same demon, an incredible alchemy occurs. Not so much around the cancer—that still most definitely sucks—but around the relationships, new and old, that pass through the white-hot fire of this experience with you. The ones who come out on the other side are the ones who will understand you inside out and will sustain you, no matter how long or short that while actually is. And they can laugh with you, no weirdness or strings attached.

What's Planet Cancer to you? What's this book? It's wisdom from the trenches. This book takes a young adult cancer patient, or a friend or family member, spouse or partner, from diagnosis all the way through treatment to readjusting in the world as someone who's been transformed by the wringer you've just gone through. And again, importantly, it's not "one person's opinion": In Planet Cancer are the battle-tested words not only of your peers, fellow residents of the Planet, but also of oncologists, of nutritionists and psychologists and even fashion designers, all of whom specialize in young adults with cancer. While there's plenty of useful medical info, you won't be reading a bunch of stats that will put you to sleep. Dr. Christian Cable, for instance—known as Dr. Disco on Planet Cancer—offers a rare glimpse into the mind of the doc as he explains how he prepares to meet a young adult cancer patient for the first time.

(Hint: He's feeling it out every bit as much as you are.)

Dr. Disco's is one of more than thirty pieces that form the cornerstone of this book: the "What It's Really Like" essays. These first-person accounts of things that happen on Planet Cancer—everything from banking sperm to wrestling with adoption to going through a clinical trial—are written by young adults who have actually been through these things. These stories are told by the people who felt it the most. And we've gotta say, they're pretty great.

You'll learn what it means when your blood counts are at certain levels and what will likely be done to you to change them. You'll learn about dating with cancer. You'll learn how to read the various tests that will determine the course of your treatment and what's good to eat (and not to) if you have mouth sores—indeed, an entire chapter is dedicated to side effects (and another to staying sane!). How to research your cancer. Do you want to research your cancer? Tips on navigating chemo treatment in the hospital. It's all in here.

You'll learn all this stuff not from someone preaching to you, but from people who drew the short straw, just like you, and came out to drop some knowledge on the other side. You'll learn a shitload, and you'll laugh too, and you'll find yourself in a great position: in charge, of both your treatment and your life. Which is a good feeling when cancer's come calling, that inconsiderate bitch.

So welcome to Planet Cancer.

We're glad you're here.

Well, not really.

But you know what we mean.

{ Remember this: It's completely understandable if your wits go AWOL upon hearing the C-word. }

Chapter One

Diagnosis

WTF? Welcome to Planet Cancer

If you're reading this, we hope you're past the shock. You know, the life-before-your-eyes rifling through everything you've ever done—cigarettes you smoked, a landfill near your hometown, the mountains of canned food you devoured over the years—anything to explain these renegade cells now doing their dirty work in your body. And the inevitable question: "Why me?"

As Reynolds Price wrote in *A Whole New Life*, "Why not?"

We know, we know—it's an annoyingly flip answer, but really it's liberating. Anybody can get cancer, and you did. It happens to nearly seventy thousand members of your peer group in the United States alone every year. Leave the shock at that and move on. Trying to assign blame, whether to the cosmos, saccharine, or the FDA, keeps you mired in worry and finger-pointing, and that's not what you need.

Here's what you do need: your wits. You're taking the wheel here; you're putting on the big-kid pants. All the doctors and nurses and drugs, the family and friends, though they have valuable roles, are movable parts in this production that, in the end, is yours.

Remember this: It's completely understandable if your wits go AWOL upon hearing the C-word. You have to get your emotional sea legs before you start dealing with anything else, like treatment. How to do this? Rely on those familiar with, first of all, your situation, and second of all, you. This means your medical team as it comes together and your family

---

Top 10 Worst Ways for an Oncologist to Break the Bad News

10. How are you set for life insurance?

9. Great news: You've got the good kind of cancer! (For all the Hodgkin's patients.)

8. So, whom do your children like to take care of them when you're not around?

7. Looks like you and I are going to be seeing a lot of each other.

6. Here, take these details about the Frequent Visitor discount in the hospital parking garage.

5. Now's your chance to lose a few extra pounds.

4. You have cancer. The nurse will fill you in. [EXITS HASTILY.]

3. I'm soooooooooo sorry.

2. Look on the bright side. Oh, wait. There is no bright side.

1. The hospital is building a new cancer center. I'd love to put you in touch with the planned-giving folks.

and friends, who will readily accommodate your primal screams as you berate the long odds that upended whatever you were doing before this tumor came along.

Whatever is the most appealing avenue for you to cope, whether it's a one-on-one discussion with a social worker at your hospital, an anonymous chat room conversation at an online resource like Planet Cancer, or tea with a long-time friend—or a combination of these—make sure you reach out. Now is not the time to retreat to your room and enter lockdown; you need support. (Also note that this state isn't unique: You will revisit this angst and frustration during treatment, so take care to note how you cope best.)

Got it? Still breathing? All right, then; let's go. As you take the first steps on this journey, here are four key points to bear in mind:

1. Be active and ask questions.

For many, being an active participant in the diagnosis and treatment process adds a sense of control to an otherwise chaotic time. Take charge, test your doctor's knowledge of your disease, and know that there's often more than one way to eradicate a tumor.

2. Get a second (third, fourth, fifth!) opinion.

It's very normal—and, in fact, advisable—to get several opinions about your disease and treatment options. Different doctors and treatment centers may suggest varying courses of action, so it only makes sense to explore your options. (Corollary: It's OK to "fire" a doctor. Your life is more important than anyone's feelings, and it's important that you be 100 percent on board with

your health-care team, and they with you.) You can even get second opinions on your pathology report, which contains your diagnosis and helps determine your suggested treatment.

3. Get organized!

We'll touch more on this in chapter 2, but suffice it to say that you're about to start amassing mountains of paper unlike anything you have ever seen. Take it from us: It's easier to set up systems to manage this avalanche of information and paperwork now rather than play catch-up a month later, as you search frantically for the document that inexplicably says you owe the hospital $267,000 for a Tylenol.

4. Rally the troops.

You will need all of your inner strength and resources during this experience, and it can be an enormous help to have others around you do some of the heavy lifting not directly related to your treatment. This may be anything from answering your phone to grocery shopping, dog walking to driving you around—whatever tasks you don't want to sap your mental or physical energy. The important thing is to learn to ask for help and to receive it gracefully. Remember that people will want to "do something" and will often be grateful for the opportunity to feel useful.

In the rest of this chapter, we'll talk about the very first things that you should think about when you receive a diagnosis of cancer. We'll get to all the other stuff—there's plenty of it—in good time, but some things need to be addressed up front, before you take one more step on your exploration of Planet Cancer.

Seeking a Second Opinion:

Always the Right Thing to Do

I wish I'd gotten a second opinion, because it turns out my first diagnosis was wrong, and I went through a few months of chemo before anyone suspected it. That's probably a one-in-a-million fluke, but if you've got even a fraction of a doubt, it's worth it to get them to send the biopsy to another lab.

—Kyle

They always say to get second opinions from different doctors, but I never thought about getting a second pathology reading. Thankfully they did it or I would have gotten the wrong chemo: The onc called me the day before I was supposed to start chemo, and I am so thankful she did.

—Lab

Asking for a second opinion is:
a) **Smart**
b) **Not rude or insulting to your doctor**
c) **Common practice**

That's not a quiz. Each answer is correct. Don't hesitate to go out there and get one more opinion (or two, or three), if only to confirm that your original doc is on target with your diagnosis and treatment recommendations. If your doctor resists, it's a huge red flag and you should think twice before sticking with him or her.

It may feel overwhelming, or like double work, to seek a second opinion when all you want to do is get started on treatment *now*. Besides, you like and trust your doc. All valid points, but remember that this is your life we're talking about here. There are very few instances (such as acute leukemia, which without exception progresses rapidly—otherwise it would be chronic leukemia) that don't allow you to hold off a little longer. After all, you've probably been misdiagnosed for months, so what's a few more days? It can't hurt to get another perspective and in some cases may make a life-altering difference in the path you take.

A second opinion from a specialist to verify your diagnosis is especially critical if your diagnosis is rare or there's not a definitive standard of care. You want to talk to someone who treats people with your disease every day, not every fifteen years.

A few things to keep in mind when you seek a second opinion:

1. Your second opinion doc should not be connected to your doctor.

Your doctor can make a referral for you and should help facilitate the process, but you should see someone outside your doctor's practice or hospital for a completely objective perspective. Get recommendations from other patients with similar diagnoses, or see whose name keeps popping up in research on your disease. (See "Researching Your Cancer" later in this chapter.)

2. Check insurance first.

Some insurance companies actually require second opinions before they'll approve some treatments. Ask whether your plan covers second opinions, and be sure to find out how much you will have to pay if the doctor you want to see is out of network. (See "Insurance" in chapter 2.)

3. **Request that all relevant records, scans, slides, and test results either be sent to the second opinion doc before your appointment or be ready for you to pick up and take with you.**

Ask your doctor's staff their process for making this happen. They may be able to do it for you, or you might have to make separate requests to every department you've been bounced to at the hospital. Whatever the case, make the request as soon as you know where you're going, ask how long it will take, and don't hesitate to be the squeaky wheel to confirm that your request is being processed (records departments are notorious for dropping the ball). You may have to pay for copies. Also be sure to ask for your pathology

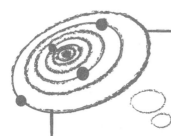

Dispatches from the Planet

Most Americans spend more time comparison shopping for a TV than they do hunting for second opinions about their cancer. The first surgeon I saw predicted that his scar would leave a slash down the back of my neck and across my throat, much like a pirate beheading. By my third surgical opinion, the scar was down to a two-inch slit in the center of my throat. You can guess which was the more experienced surgeon and who I went with.

Fast-forward two rounds of treatment and five years later: A stash of new tumors cropped up in my neck. My doc and I read the biopsy report together, scratching our heads. The size and locations didn't make sense.

"The pathologist was probably chowing on a sandwich and flirting on the phone with his girlfriend while he wrote the report," he said. "I'll ask for a second opinion from a different pathologist." Who knew you can get a second opinion from not

just a surgeon or oncologist, but from a pathologist too?

I was on a roll. Yes, I was mid-cancer career with an established team of doctors, but I wanted a fresh perspective before I dove into round two of surgery. I crammed a second, third, and fourth opinion at three different hospitals into one afternoon. I revealed to each doctor my itinerary, expecting they would be pissed off and defensive and give me the you're-a-high-maintenance-patient eye roll. Instead, they were fired up by my oncology road show, wanted to learn from the opinions of their colleagues, and helped me understand why some of them had differing approaches. Going under the knife a second time sucked, but at least I had peace of mind knowing I had found the best care possible.

—Kairol Rosenthal

report. Bringing your records can save you from unnecessarily repeating tests that have been performed already.

> Researchers at Johns Hopkins Hospital found that 2 percent of all pathology reports at large medical centers are incorrect; such missteps on the front end can lead to misdiagnoses and inappropriate treatments.

4. If you get conflicting advice from the second opinion, get a third. Keep going until you feel comfortable with the diagnosis and treatment recommendations. It's worth it!

The point is to be comfortable with your doctor and your treatment. If you like your doctor, it's perfectly acceptable to bring other treatment options back to him or her.

My wife, Sally, was first diagnosed with breast cancer at twenty-nine. After telling her that it was probably nothing and that she was too young to have breast cancer, Sally's OB-GYN sent her to a general surgeon for a biopsy. The doctor decided to tell Sally she had cancer while he was performing the biopsy!

He then said to me within earshot of my wife, "Your wife has cancer. I will remove her breast on Monday, and you won't have any children." I thanked him, told him we'd call him, and got the heck out of that hospital.

Through a combination of coincidence and good luck, we found Dr. Freya Schnabel. She gave us a different perspective and reassured Sally. Yes, she would need surgery, chemo, and radiation, but, she added, "You will buy economy-size shampoo again." Last month during a checkup we recalled that proclamation made seventeen years ago, almost to the day.

Sally's surgery was more invasive due to the error made by the first doctor, who had cut into the tumor rather than removing the entire lump.

She volunteered for a protocol that increased the amount of chemo given in a shorter amount of time. This was followed by six weeks of radiation. The chemo treatments were strong, and doctors feared that they would jeopardize Sally's reproductive organs. When that didn't happen, the doctors thought that since her cancer was estrogen- and progesterone-positive, becoming pregnant would increase the chances of a recurrence.

We waited five years. After more tests, discussions, heart-to-hearts, etc., doctors gave us the OK. In 2000 Sally gave birth to our little miracle child, Christina. Doctor Schnabel still claims that it was one of the biggest moments of her career.

This experience was of enormous help when my mother was diagnosed with cancer in 2001. I knew how to react and got my mother to the proper doctors who would help ensure the best chance of her survival. A second opinion is vital and gives patients peace of mind in knowing that their illness is being treated properly.

—Anthony MJ Colistra

Fertility

To the surprise of my oncologist, my most recent CT and PET scans suggest that the cancer may be back. If I have relapsed, then I will need a stem cell transplant, and after that, I will most likely be sterile. So I am very, very glad that I gathered embryos when I did.

—Andrea U

Sadly, young adult cancer patients too often find their fertility gone before being able to do anything about it. That is, many aren't told to bank sperm or harvest eggs while they still can; chemo, surgery, or radiation rolls in and renders young adult reproductive business-as-usual impossible.

We're telling you now: Do it! Ask about every possible fertility option before your treatment starts. If your chemo needed to begin yesterday—if it did begin yesterday—ask anyway. If you're twenty-three and you think you'll never want kids, *ask anyway!* Doctors and fertility clinics should work with you to harvest eggs or bank sperm as quickly as possible, if it is possible. And even if you can't do anything, at least you won't look back in five years and wonder,

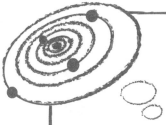

Dispatches from the Planet

I had to get a checkup PET/CT and was scheduling it over the phone. The woman (she sounded very young) asked me if I could be pregnant and when my last period was. I told her that I lost my period in 2005 due to my chemo. She said, "Boy, you're lucky." I guess she realized she may have made a mistake saying that, seeing as how I am only twenty-nine and have no kids. I find it funny how some people don't realize that there are so many more things to worry about even after you're in remission. While I don't mind missing the monthly visit from Aunt Flo, I wish I could have had the opportunity to have kids of my own before I got sick.

—Emily Olsen

I was twenty-six when I was diagnosed with Stage IV non-Hodgkin's lymphoma, one month after my high school sweetheart had proposed. The oncologist informed me of possible infertility, and also of possible menopause, after receiving six rounds of CHOP chemotherapy. (See sidebar on page 7.) I was referred to a local fertility specialist, and my oncologist gave me one month to delay treatment. They acted fast. We produced twenty-six embryos with my fiancé's sperm and my retrieved eggs.

—Tiffany Hoover

What if . . . . There's absolutely nothing to put before learning about your fertility options and putting what you learn into action, if humanly—and medically—possible.

The go-to resource for every cancer patient exploring fertility preservation is Fertile Hope (www.fertilehope.org). An initiative of **LIVESTRONG,** Lance Armstrong's foundation, Fertile Hope provides comprehensive fertility information and assistance, from a fertility options calculator to discounted services for fertility preservation.

> **CHOP is a chemo combination of: C (cyclo-phosphamide); H (hydroxydoxorubicin, a.k.a. Adriamycin, a.k.a. the "Red Devil"); O (Oncovin, trade name for vincristine); P (prednisone, a steroid, and, some would argue, the worst part).**

What it's really like to . . .
Have Your Eggs Harvested, or Persephone Wears a White Coat

by Lauren Rachel Ainsworth

Like most young women, I took my fertility for granted. Forget babysitting; I hated kids so much that I quit a lifeguarding job in high school after two weeks because I couldn't stand dealing with the brats all day, even from the safety of a ten-foot stand. I even went as far as to ask my gynecologist a couple of years later if she would perform a tubal ligation because I felt that I lacked the "maternal gene" and I was tired of taking birth control pills. She refused.

Apparently things change when you hear the words, "You have cancer." When I was diagnosed with Hodgkin's lymphoma in 2004, one of the first questions I asked my oncologist was "How will this affect my fertility?" Instantaneously, I had come to the realization that my evolution-ary value would be compromised, and without my consent. However unacceptable this was, I was not given any options for fertility preservation at the time, so I plunged into chemotherapy with nothing more than the hope that my ovaries would withstand the rigors of treatment.

Six months later, I was in remission. My ovarian function was slightly compromised by the treatments I received, but it didn't bother me too much. I was still young at twenty-two, and I had more important things to worry about, like work, school, and health insurance—until the cancer came back three years later.

I was given a 90 percent guarantee that I would have no ovarian function following the treatment of my relapse, which was to include more chemotherapy, radiation, and a stem cell transplant. Luckily, the relapse was caught early, and although I was again symptomatic, my doctor encouraged me to pursue fertility preservation options. I researched these options and, thanks to a wealth of information and financial assistance provided by Fertile Hope, decided on egg (oocyte) freezing.

On my first visit to the reproductive endocrinologist, blood was taken to determine my FSH (follicle stimulating hormone) level, and the first of many trans-vaginal ultrasounds (also affectionately known as "probings") was performed. The baseline FSH and ultrasound are very important. They help your doctor determine how fertile you are, as well as what medications and dosages to give you based on these measurements. I showed about half the amount of follicles expected for a twenty-five-year-old, and my FSH was elevated, but my doctor and I decided that pursuing this option was still worth it, even if I didn't produce very many eggs to freeze.

The egg retrieval process takes about three weeks. The first week, you take birth control pills to suppress the ovaries and prepare them for stimulation. The second and third weeks involve constant ovarian stimulation through the use of injectable hormones. You give yourself four stimulating medications over the course of the two-week cycle in the comfort of your own bathroom. When I started giving myself these drugs, it felt almost as if I'd become my own compounding pharmacy—my cabinets and refrigerator were stocked with two full bags of fertility drugs worth more than a gold Rolex, and I mixed and injected them nightly. All the drugs were injected subcutaneously with the tiniest of needles, into the stubborn, crunch-resistant layer of fat just below my belly button.

When the stimulation cycle began, I had to go to the doctor's office every other day for an early-morning probing and blood work in order to monitor my progress. These appointments usually took less than an hour, and I ended up saving plenty of money that would've otherwise been spent at Starbucks; nothing wakes you up in the morning quite like a nice, cold, vigorous ultrasound probing.

Surprisingly, the side effects of the fertility medications were minimal. I was both shocked and dismayed that I hadn't grown fangs and retractable claws by the end of the treatment cycle. The stereotypical bitchiness and emotional liability associated with fertility treatments proved to be simply the workings of talented Hollywood writers. It wasn't until two hours after the last drug, a hefty dose of the pregnancy hormone human chorionic gonadotropin, given thirty-six hours before the retrieval surgery, that I began crying uncontrollably, but that only lasted an hour or two. There was minimal pain and very little weight gain associated with the stimulation medication. I could feel the presence of my orange-sized ovaries by the end of the cycle, but only when I walked around.

Versed and fentanyl are combined regularly when patients require IV sedation. During IV sedation, you enter a sleepy, dreamlike state, but without needing respirators or anesthesiologists. Fentanyl is a very strong pain medication, and Versed is a sedative. When they are combined and administered via IV drip, it feels as if you've had about six margaritas with amnesia instead of salt on the rim.

The actual egg retrieval procedure was painless, thanks to my very skilled physician and copious amounts of Versed and fentanyl. Eggs are removed from mature ovarian follicles during outpatient surgery. Basically, the eggs are sucked out of the follicles individually through a needle that is inserted into the cervix, through the wall of the uterus, and into the ovary. They are then rapidly frozen and stored for future use. I felt very little pain following the surgery, and I was able to resume my usual weekend activities the next day, which consisted of short trips from my bed to the bathroom and kitchen during the commercials of an *America's Next Top Model* rerun-watching marathon.

Overall, the process was quick, easy, and relatively painless, especially compared to cancer treatment. The hardest part for me was sitting alone in the waiting room at the fertility clinic every other day, ever so aware that not only was I single and ten years younger than every woman and doting husband waiting with me, but also that I would not walk out of the clinic pregnant and happy. Rather, I would leave and go a mile down the street to M.D. Anderson and fight for my life—again. The best part of the whole process, however, was knowing when I'd left that seven frozen chances at motherhood, seven tiny Eggsicles, would be waiting there for me to return after I'd won that fight.

Note: *Egg harvesting is still considered "investigational" by the American Society of Clinical Oncology, meaning that, though the procedure has worked successfully in some instances, it is far from being perfected, and its success cannot be guaranteed.*

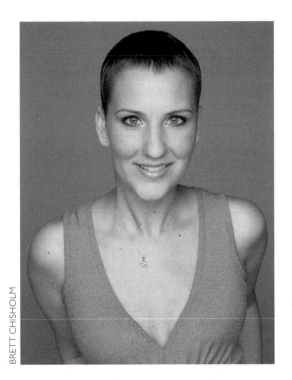

BRETT CHISHOLM

Guides to the Planet

Lauren Rachel Ainsworth, now twenty-six, was diagnosed with Hodgkin's lymphoma in 2004. Her pastimes include extensive PubMed searches, overflowing the mailbox at M.D. Anderson Cancer Center with suggestions and complaints, hitting on single male physicians, critiquing hospital cuisine, and playing the cello. Rachel resides in her hometown, Houston, and is pursuing graduate study in epidemiology at the University of Texas School of Public Health.

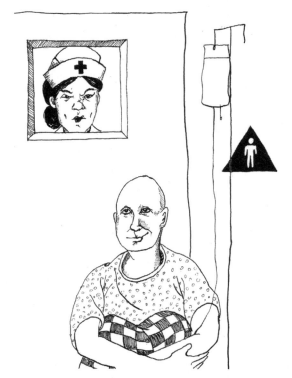

Top 10 Ways to Break the Ice with Your Nurse

10. Fill bedpan with chocolate pudding and salsa; whistle the *Mission: Impossible* theme as she carries it away.

9. Call her "stewardess."

8. Try to convince her of your firm conviction that your tumor is the karmic by-product of "all those kids I ate."

7. Lock her in the bathroom; insist that she refer to you as "Warden."

6. Act baffled when she enters to minister to you and say: "They told me I had a prostrate dancer."

5. Sew your right hand to your lips and laugh whenever she's around—oblivious to your dementia, she'll of course think you're cute and have a funny little secret.

4. Ask her if she wants to play "Find the caduceus."

3. Strategically place a copy of *Hustler* sticking out from under your mattress, your subscription label clearly visible. After all, they love readers.

2. Demand that the doctor tell you why the night shift nurses dress in snowsuits and shout at you in Icelandic.

1. Constantly compliment her on the "hot nurse costume" she's wearing.

Guides to the Planet

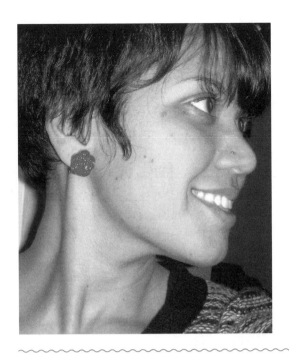

Nadyne Wood, who contributed the illustrations accompanying the Top 10 lists in the book, is an illustrator and a wife; equally important, she is a cancer survivor: She has overcome the brain tumor she was diagnosed with in 2004. As a result, she has found great gifts in a situation that seemed so dark and difficult. She believes the experience has made her a better person and a better artist. See more of Nadyne's illustrations at www.nadynewood.com. Nadyne lives in Brooklyn, New York, with her husband, Darby, and three pets.

What it's really like to . . .

Bank Sperm

by Justin Sullivan

What's it really like to bank sperm? Uncomfortable. When I banked, I wasn't allowed to use any sort of lubrication. Not even a little spit. The only good thing that has ever come from spinning dry wood is fire. Someday I hope to add kids to this very short list.

I walked into the bank about 9:30 in the morning. I was ready. I had hyped myself up for the event. I was like a fighter entering the ring for the championship belt. My opponent . . . well, my opponent was a five-foot-two, ninety-year-old lady who sat at the front desk. She had more wrinkles on her face than I did on my balls. All my preparation, all my courage, all my hope diminished in an instant. I quickly realized that this wasn't going to be easy.

The office was about six feet by ten feet with a door that sat right next to the old woman's desk. She led me through the door into this tiny bathroom. There was a toilet, a sink, enough room to stand between them, and a basket with a magazine. Yes, one magazine. It had been so worked over that I could not bring myself to touch it. I had to do this one freestyle. Since I'd waited until two days before chemo started, this was it. This was possibly my last chance to make a baby. She handed me a cup, turned around, and closed the door.

The weight of the moment settled on my shoulders. It was heavy. Performance under pressure at its finest. I began to imagine myself in some wonderful place with a beautiful woman who had on a long silky robe with nothing underneath, and she sang a seductive song with a raspy voice that went something like, "How's it going in there?"

It was a mess. And not the good kind of mess you would associate with making babies. But it's what I had to do. Rub one out for the future of my namesake. There's no question it was the smartest thing I have ever done when it comes to my treatment. I didn't think so at the time. But I hope that doing my thing as the little old lady stood guard will lead to one of life's greatest gifts. Children.

In short, what's it like? It's uncomfortable, embarrassing, sad, a little painful, and yet very reassuring all at the same time. I would do it again in a heartbeat. But next time I would bring my own magazine.

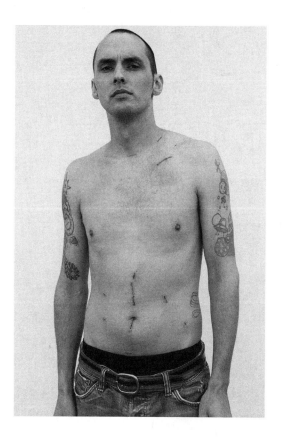

Guides to the Planet

Justin Sullivan was diagnosed with Stage II Hodgkin's disease at age twenty-eight on April 2, 2004, the day he graduated from film school. In 2008, at age thirty-three, Justin went through his second stem cell transplant at National Institutes of Health. Six months later, he moved to Brooklyn, New York, where he worked in fashion photography and continued to battle cancer. A constant researcher, he kept his oncologists at NIH and then Sloan Kettering on their toes as he suggested new treatment regimens and protocols. Even as cancer ravaged his body, Justin continued to celebrate life's bright moments with a hip-shaking boogie! Justin returned to his native Texas for the last chapter of his life, and spent his last days with the love of his life, family, friends, and his teenage daughter. A fighter to the end, on December 12, 2009, Justin Sullivan lost his battle with cancer.

If Your Fertility Is Compromised or You Must Start Treatment Immediately

If your situation is such that you must start treatment lickety-split and don't have time to preserve eggs or bank sperm, don't panic! All hope isn't lost; you can still become a parent. Focus on what you need to with your treatment; you'll have multiple options later. When later comes—six to twelve months post-treatment—have your fertility tested. You'll fall into one of four categories:

1. **Your fertility will be normal.**

2. **You'll have temporary infertility.** Early onset of menopause related to treatment may not always be permanent. Some women's fertility does return, although women who have had chemotherapy will eventually enter menopause sooner than they would have otherwise.

3. **You'll have compromised fertility.** Your uterus has been removed, for example, or your sperm production has been impaired. In this case you'll need to work with a doctor to figure out your best options.

4. **You'll be infertile/sterile.** Based on your fertility test results, you'll take one (or more) of many different paths. What you should remember, however, is that no matter your fertility status, you have a ton of options. Here are just a few to consider:

   - **Donor eggs, donor embryos, or donor sperm.**

   - **Assisted reproductive technologies:** This term covers a lot of different things a reproductive doctor can help you with, such as, for women, in vitro fertilization (IVF) and gestational surrogacy (a woman carries a baby for you using either her own eggs or donor eggs—the baby can have genetic ties to you but it doesn't have to). For men, if you didn't bank sperm pretreatment and are infertile, testicular sperm extraction is a possibility: Doctors can remove residual sperm from your testicles and use that in IVF. (Caveat: This one is really expensive, and insurance generally does not cover it.)

   - **Adoption:** It's always an option for anyone (even if you're fertile!). Adoption can be challenging if you have a negative medical history (see "Family Planning . . . Finally" in chapter 7), and many adoption agencies keep this type of "negative" information close to their chest. For example, China has a law that cancer survivors can't adopt Chinese babies, so don't pursue that route and waste your time and energy.

Researching Your Cancer: Do You Wanna Go There?

I remember having an appointment with my oncologist where I brought research that I wanted to review with him. I don't think he'd had that happen before.

—KATE

There are pros and cons to digging deep and learning everything you can about your cancer. They all pretty much relate to whether or not you believe the old saw, "What you don't know won't hurt you."

With that in mind, tell your doctor up front—as well as anyone doing research for you—just how much detail you want about survival statistics and your prognosis. Some people want every possible number; some don't want a single one. It's your prerogative. Below is a list to help you decide what you do want to know. Much of it comes to us with the permission of Steve Dunn's CancerGuide, a no-frills, up-to-date, compendious but easily digested online repository of cancer information (www.cancerguide.org), designed to help patients perform research as simply as possible.

Pros of Researching Your Cancer

1. It Could Save Your Life.

- No doctor can keep up with every promising new development for every type of cancer. As a patient, you only have to research one kind of cancer and one situation: yours. You have a lot more time than any doctor to spend on your case, and you might find a treatment that your doctor doesn't know about that could save your life.

- Some physicians don't keep up well and, if you have such a doctor, even a small amount of research can reveal a standard treatment with a higher success rate than what your doctor is proposing.

- If you're an HMO member, know this: The less care an HMO gives, and the less often it refers patients outside its network, the more profit it makes. So there exists, at times, a conflict between your best interests and those of your HMO. This doesn't mean that HMOs always shortchange their patients; some patients receive excellent treatment. However, given the push for profits, it can't hurt to assume that HMOs are less likely to tell their patients about promising new treatments or clinical trials, particularly if these treatments or trials are not available within their network. In this situation, a little research could save your life.

- If your cancer is rare, your doctor probably has little or no experience treating it. Through research, you might find an expert on your disease and whatever is known about its treatment.

2. It Salvages Some Control.

- Invasive or toxic treatments and procedures that you don't fully understand can make you feel as if everything happening to you is beyond your control. Understanding your medical treatment can be a powerful antidote to feeling helpless and hopeless, and will also help you do everything possible to make it successful.

- Through research you learn success rates, side effects, and prognoses more thoroughly than you normally would during a doctor's appointment. Armed with knowledge of your cancer and its various treatment options, you can discuss the whys of any decisions you come to on your own with your doctor. And if you make a mistake in interpreting what you find, your doctor will have a chance to correct it.

Cons of Researching Your Cancer

1. Medical Research Can Be Difficult and Intimidating.

Plowing through the thick jargon of technical medical literature isn't easy, but don't assume that to do it successfully you need an upper-level science degree. Determination goes a long way, and when you're fighting for your life, motivation is high. A possible solution: If reading densely written technical reports isn't your thing, maybe someone you know would be willing to help. Most friends and relatives wish they could do something to help but don't know what that might be. Research could be just the thing!

2. You Might Make the Wrong Decision.

If you stubbornly lone-wolf your research, you could misinterpret what you read and make a bad decision. The solution: Be sure to include your doctor in your thinking and decision-making, and to weigh his or her input carefully.

3. You Will Confront the Statistics.

This can be difficult. As Steve Dunn wrote: "I was diagnosed with metastatic disease only four days after I read a paper that gave the three-year survival for my cancer with metastatic disease as only 4 percent. Knowing this dismal statistic was terribly, terribly difficult, but I was able to realize that 4 percent is not 0 percent, and also that new treatments could raise these odds."

Understanding what the statistics really mean, however, can actually help you salvage hope from despair. Let's say you've heard a poor prognosis for your cancer. The median survival rate is one year—pretty crappy, one

would assume. The average person likely thinks, "What? By this time next year I'm out?"

Wrong. Figuring out exactly what a median survival rate of a year means can be a key first step toward entering treatment on your own terms, with the proper mind-set, and not falling mistakenly into doom and gloom.

Let's break it down: The median is the middle representative of a group. It's not the aver-

> So think about it and don't forget it: You are a statistic of exactly one. Don't enter your treatment in a state of shock or resignation.

age but is rather the number below and above which half the numbers occur.

In the following illustration (it's called a histogram, so you know, but don't go to sleep!), you can see what a median of one year means: Half the patients died within one year of the date of diagnosis; the half that survived beyond that first year, however, lasted far beyond—out to twenty to thirty years.

Stephen Jay Gould, a Harvard scientist and a fine writer, was diagnosed with mesothelioma in 1982 and learned that the median survival rate for his cancer was eight months. He went to the library at Harvard, read everything about mesothelioma, and came out in much better spirits.

In a brilliant essay called "The Median Isn't the Message" (available online at www.cancer guide.org/median_not_msg.html), Gould points out that the eight-month median for mesothe-

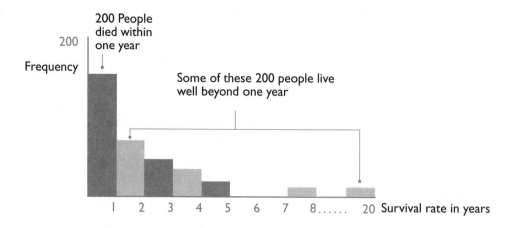

200

Frequency

200 People died within one year

Some of these 200 people live well beyond one year

1 2 3 4 5 6 7 8 . . . . . . 20 Survival rate in years

lioma is "right-skewed," meaning that some of those with mesothelioma who didn't die before eight months likely stretched their lives far beyond the median. Put another way, on the right, the graph could stretch out for years and years, and in fact did.

What makes a patient outlast the median? Gould's answer: "Match people with the same cancer for age, class, health, socioeconomic status, and, in general, those with positive attitudes, with a strong will and purpose for living, with commitment to struggle, with an active response to aiding their own treatment and not just a passive acceptance of anything doctors say, tend to live longer." He knew he fell into this group and had an informed conviction that he'd outlive the median survival rate for his cancer.

Matching age is particularly important for young adults: Consider that many of these statistics come from studies conducted primarily on people your grandparents' age, with all the accompanying infirmities that can affect outcomes.

So think about it and don't forget it: You are

a statistic of exactly one. Don't enter your treatment in a state of shock or resignation. Enter it in control, enter it informed, and enter it as you do the rest of your life—with a young person's zest for living. As for Gould, he left the Planet, sanguine disposition intact, in 2002. He died from a disease entirely unrelated to the mesothelioma he had fully recovered from.

A final note: Reading out-of-date statistics can make you think things are worse than they are because treatment may have improved. Never rely on old data!

4. There Might Not Be Any Better Treatment Available.

It is quite possible that, even after a lot of time and effort, you will find no better treatment than the one your doctor recommended in the first place. While this may be disappointing if you were searching for a magic bullet, there is something to be said for knowing that your doctor is recommending the best treatment available, which can increase your confidence.

How to Research Your Cancer

We could write a separate book on the arcane ins and outs of searching PDQ (www.cancer.gov/cancertopics/pdq/cancerdatabase), and PubMed (www.ncbi.nlm.nih.gov/PubMed/), but we figure that the most useful thing to do is give you some general principles and guidelines to steer you safely through the wild west of Internet cancer research.

A few points to keep in mind as you dive in:

• Knowledge is power.

• Every person's cancer experience is unique.

• A healthy dose of skepticism is good.

PDQ

(www.cancer.gov/cancertopics/pdq/cancer database) stands for Physician Data Query, a cancer database compiled by the National Cancer Institute. It includes basic information, treatment summaries (both patient and physician versions), and a registry of thousands of clinical trials from around the world.

PubMed

(www.ncbi.nlm.nih.gov/PubMed/) is an online service of the U.S. National Library of Medicine. It provides links to millions of journal articles and other biomedical resources.

Before You Start

To keep your research focused, make sure you are prepared *before* you start searching. Have at your fingertips all the info you have been given by your doctors, such as the specific diagnosis, stage, grade, and site of your cancer. Even better, write down specific questions that you want to have answered. For example:

What is the standard of care for my diagnosis?

Are there any clinical trials available that take a new approach toward treating my disease? (See also "Clinical Trials" in chapter 3.)

Who is the leading authority on my diagnosis?

Are there any support resources available for people in my circumstance?

WHERE TO LOOK

There are a gazillion Web sites out there. The ones that will probably end up being most useful to you will more than likely fall into one of the main categories below, requiring different levels of skepticism, based on the expertise of the person posting the information. The gold standard is evidence-based research that has been peer-reviewed and published in a medical journal.

Commercial: This primarily means pharmaceutical companies, especially if you're looking for drug-specific information. While pharma conducts a great deal of valuable research, it's also worth remembering that it is in the business of selling drugs. Quality research—pharma or otherwise—will be published in a credible medical journal.

Medical organizations: Medical professional societies, such as the American Society of Clinical Oncology (ASCO), often have helpful information for health-care professionals and patients.

Government: Federal and state governments offer a variety of resources ranging from clinical trials information to financial assistance programs.

Nonprofit: There are nongovernmental organizations focused on almost every aspect of the cancer experience: disease-specific information, lifestyle challenges, financial assistance, emotional support, and more. Some are great and credible, some not so much. Look at how current the information is, whether they have credible medical advisors, who is behind the site or organization, and how they are funded. Sites that are too obviously a reflection of one person's biases—nonprofit or not—should be avoided or taken with a grain of salt.

Personal: Sites started and run by individuals can be very helpful, but be aware that they can be all over the credibility map, ranging from personal blogs to comprehensive informational resources.

Start with an Overview

Dip your toes in the research waters by starting with recognized, reputable sites that offer layman-focused summaries of cancer in general and your type in particular. Visit their links pages for direction on where to go next as you drill down and focus your search. Some good ones for starters:

- American Cancer Society (www.cancer.org).

- National Cancer Institute (www.cancer.gov): Review the patient versions of the PDQ cancer information summaries—these layman's ver-

sions of the summaries are easier to understand than doctors' writings, which will be more full of jargon that will be harder to understand, especially if you're just starting to research.

- OncoLink (www.oncolink.org): Cancer information from the University of Pennsylvania.

- Cancer.net: The patient-focused site of the American Society of Clinical Oncology.

- MacMillan Cancer Support (www.macmillan .org.uk): A UK-based organization with easy-to-navigate cancer information.

- MedLine Plus (www.nlm.nih.gov/medline plus/).

- For disease-specific searches, go to sites of large national nonprofit organizations focused on the individual diagnosis, such as the Lymphoma Research Foundation (www .lymphoma.org) or the American Brain Tumor Association (www.abta.org).

Dig a Little Deeper

Once you have a general handle on your situation and start becoming more conversant with the lingo, you may want to dive deeper into the medical literature for more detailed information, such as evaluating treatment options or exploring clinical trials, side effect information, or outcomes data. There are a few exceptionally powerful medical databases that offer a gold mine of biomedical articles and citations. Start with the FAQ or Help section of these sites to familiarize yourself with how they work and how to manipulate the keywords and combinations that will yield the best results.

- **National Cancer Institute** (www.cancer.gov): Dive into the professional versions of those PDQ cancer information summaries.

- **PubMed** (www.ncbi.nlm.nih.gov/PubMed/): The mother lode. A service of the National Institutes of Health and the U.S. National Library of Medicine that gives free access to millions of citations of biomedical articles from the MedLine database and various journals. Definitely do your homework on how to use PubMed before diving straight in. It will save you time, frustration, and confusion.

- **ClinicalTrials.gov:** This site, maintained by the National Institutes of Health, is a list of clinical trials occurring worldwide, including information about their purpose, who may participate in the trials, and the relevant contact information.

Keep Going

As Steve Dunn's CancerGuide says, "Researching the literature is not a single path that proceeds straight from initial question to final answer. It is actually more like a cycle. Initial questions lead to references to the medical literature, which lead to papers, which lead to more references, and more questions. . . . "

It takes patience and persistence to do research, but what could be more important? Just stay focused, take copious notes, and bounce your findings off your doctor. Be wary, however, of the paralytic effect of researching, where you continually second-guess yourself. It's a fine line, but one that's important to draw. Research until you feel that you've amassed enough evidence to make an informed decision, discuss with your key advisors, decide, then—very important—turn the computer off and go do something nice for yourself.

Top 10 Signs That a Web Site Is a BIG FAT SCAM

10. Contact information is: MrAnonymous@anon.xrtnws.co.kz

9. "This is not a scam."

8. Credibility comes from: "As seen on Geraldo!"

7. Last updated in 1993.

6. "Based on scientific principles that are thousands of years old" (ancient Chinese secret).

5. LOTS OF CAPITAL LETTERS and "punctuation"!!!

4. Scientific evidence is all presented in made-for-TV-movie stories.

3. It wants you to send in money before revealing any of its secrets.

2. "Money-back guarantee! NO QUESTIONS ASKED!"

1. The powerful medical/pharmaceutical/government establishment is trying to suppress the work of the discoverer.

{ Confessions of a PubMed Addict }

by Lauren Rachel Ainsworth

Hi, my name is Rachel, and I'm a PubMed addict. ("Hi, Rachel.")

Like many addictions, it all started innocently enough. I was a Hodgkin's disease survivor at the apex of life, with two good years of clinical research experience under my belt. Cancer had knocked me down, but not out, during my senior year of college, and from then on I had known my calling: kicking cancer's ass through the study of public health; specifically, epidemiology, the study of the distribution and determinants of disease.

I began my postgraduate program in August of my twenty-fifth year. One month later, I had my three-year post-treatment follow-up exams. I was so immersed in learning the basics of my new field that I didn't even worry about the results of my tests until the doctors refused to give me the results over the phone or by fax. When my doctor finally gave word that my PET scan was positive and my blood work wonky—ominous signs that the scourge had returned—he told me not to worry. "Concentrate on school for now," he said, "Let's take another look when your semester is over, and we'll repeat the scans then." Concentrate I did.

Fully equipped with a fresh set of high-level research skills, unlimited access to hundreds of millions of full-text electronic journal articles, a handful of M.D. and Ph.D. colleagues and friends (including my neighbor, the hematology post-doc, and my best friend, the breast cancer researcher), a borderline-clinical anxiety disorder,

and enough ADHD meds to give an elephant a heart attack, I went straight to work.

I was being trained to understand medical research, to review, synthesize, and critique existing research, and to conduct my own research. I knew which study designs to look for, the number of participants and statistics needed to make the results significant, how to spot confounding variables, the works. I knew what most of the terms meant already, and when I didn't understand the cancer jargon, I gave myself honorary degrees in hematology and pharmacology.

Fueled by raw fear, my addiction to PubMed (the National Institutes of Health electronic database) overcame me faster than mouth sores appear during a melphalan drip. If treatment decisions were to be made, I showed up to the clinic with manila folders full of copied, collated, stapled, and highlighted articles in one hand, and a double latte in the other, eyes bloodshot from the all-nighter spent scouring the databases the night before. Imagine WebMD on crystal meth and steroids, secured by a binder clip.

At first, the doctors were patient, but, understandably, their tolerance of my second-guessing, often smart-alecky antics waned. It's not that they didn't appreciate my thirst for knowledge or my being an active participant in my own treatment decisions. They recognized, long before I did, that my refusal to relinquish control had gone well out of control. Eventually my entire team (psychiatric service included) surprised me with an intervention worthy of the A&E documentary series while I, a captive audience in my hospital bed, sobbed and complained about the Phase I trial they had presented to me hours before.

Somewhere along the way, amid the fog of chemo brain, the Ativan and Dilaudid cocktails, and the trauma of the realization that I was insulting and awfully arrogant to disrespect their expertise to such a severe degree, I admitted that I had a problem. I will admit wholeheartedly that that first step was the most important one.

Relinquishing control was synonymous with moving on with treatment, and moving on with life. My physicians still might fantasize about choking me with my own highlighter during our question-and-answer sessions, but they hide it well now and seem even more forthcoming with their answers now that we have worked on a fine balance of mutual respect and admiration of each other's knowledge.

Misdiagnosis

When the lump first appeared in my neck, my mom took me to the doctor, and after he took my blood, felt the lump, etc., my mom said to him, "Could it be Hodgkin's? A boy in her class had the same thing last year, with the same symptoms." He was flat-out convinced it wasn't. He handed me some antibiotics and sent me on my way. We went back to him a year later, and he told me some people just have lumps in their neck. It wasn't until I had been sick for nearly three years that I was finally diagnosed! With Hodgkin's! My mom had been right all along.

—Jenifer

Unfortunately, young adults (defined by the National Cancer Institute as fifteen- to thirty-nine-year-olds) are statistically more likely to experience a misdiagnosis compared with older people or children. This doesn't mean doctors are incompetent or evil. Face it: You're a statistical outlier. You are to Planet Cancer what Pauly Shore is to Hollywood. Which is to say: Who, including your doctor—not to mention yourself—really expected to see you here?

Sometimes we forget that doctors are people too. We cling to an irrational idea that doctors should always know exactly what's going on with our bodies, as if under our skin there's a world as cut-and-dried, as black and white and easily diagnosed and cured as the two-dimensional cartoon figure in medicine commercials—the one with a circular stomach whose pain is signified, as Jerry Seinfeld has pointed out, by tiny lightning bolts.

Though both Hodgkin's and non-Hodgkin's lymphoma, or NHL, are lymphomas that attack your immune system, they're treated differently. The difference between the two lymphomas involves the presence of Reed-Sternberg cells: Hodgkin's has them, NHL doesn't. For every incidence of Hodgkin's, there are about five of NHL. The fifth-most common cancer in the United States, NHL affects slightly more men than women.

> Improvements in cancer survival rates for young adults have lagged behind the gains made for their older and younger counter-parts. In some subsets, there has been no improvement in thirty years.

Obviously this isn't the case. Doctors aren't always right. Egregious cases of misdiagnosis may deserve legal recourse or a filing with your state's medical board. If you want to pursue legal action, the most efficient way is to contact the largest malpractice firm in your area and ask to speak with an attorney who specializes in your specific diagnosis. (If the firm doesn't have one, move on to the next firm—the attorney's familiarity/case history with your type of cancer is most important here.)

If you just want some comeuppance visited on your doctor, contact your state's medical board. It'll be anonymous and there's a chance that your doctor won't hear about it, but rest assured that if the medical board gets several complaints about the same doctor, it should at least prompt an investigation.

For the good docs who just plain missed it, why not send a letter or an e-mail to let him or her know what the correct diagnosis was? Review your symptoms, share what test finally confirmed cancer and some stats on young adult cancer, and encourage your doc not to dismiss out of hand the possibility of cancer in another young adult.

Granted, it won't change your own situation, but it could prevent the future misdiagnosis of another young adult patient. And hey, a strongly worded letter is a great place to vent anger or bitterness that you may have brewing. Then, unless you're taking more drastic measures, you can close the door on that issue and get on with the business at hand—saving your ass.

Following are a few examples plucked from the Planet that show both the fallibility of doctors and the resilience of young adult patients; you can find many more on the Planet Cancer Web site (www.planetcancer.org). Seriously, we could not make some of this stuff up if we tried.

> A 2005 article published by *HealthDay News* cited misdiagnosis rates of 2 to 9 percent in gynecological cases and 5 to 12 percent in nongynecological cases. It's worth noting that this means that cancer is not diagnosed—not that there is a false diagnosis of cancer.

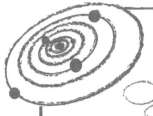

Dispatches from the Planet

Shanti's Hodgkin's disease presented with a cough, and she was misdiagnosed with:

1. Tuberculosis
2. Asthma
3. Bronchitis
4. And the kicker . . . SARS. ("Since I had just gotten back from the Philippines. . . . Gotta laugh at doctors," she writes. "Gotta laugh so you don't cry.")

WillieB's diagnostic roller coaster lasted from December 2004 to January 2006:

1. All manner of intestinal infections.
2. A gall bladder surgery that was supposed to fix everything.
3. Diagnosed with metastatic adenitis.
4. An appendectomy that was supposed to fix everything.
5. Diagnosed with kidney stones.
6. Stage IV aggressive large B cell lymphoma.

"I now have a whole new set of doctors," WillieB writes, "and try not to remember the first group ever existed."

What it's really like to . . .
Be Misdiagnosed

by William Patrick Tandy

I had a persistent low-grade fever—ninety-nine, one hundred degrees—and a dull pain in my neck. I hadn't slept well in nearly a week, in spite of the ulcer-inducing amount of ibuprofen I had ingested. Unable to make a timely appointment with my primary-care physician (PCP), one day I left work early and, on the recommendation of a coworker, went straight to a walk-in clinic. There

I was diagnosed with "cat-scratch fever." Right, I thought. Are you sure it isn't rockin' pneumonia brought on by complications from an untreated case of boogie-woogie flu?

I learned, however, that cat-scratch fever is a very real thing, and its symptoms are not unlike those of mononucleosis. And, as with mono, there's little more to do to treat it than eat well and rest.

Three weeks later I awoke at night with terrible headaches, and the dull pain in my neck had developed into a full-bore throb and had become unsettlingly swollen. I returned to the walk-in clinic. The attending physician—a different one now—expressed visible concern. "A normal lymph node is about the size of your thumbnail, maybe a centimeter," she said. "You've got one in your neck that's about seven centimeters." As it so happened, she knew my PCP personally. "Go see her," said the doc. "Now."

Because of my age and the fact that non-Hodgkin's statistically strikes more elderly patients, no one, I'm sure, thought that that might be my problem. Nevertheless, all of the doctors involved handled my case with professionalism and empathy. Consequently, in less than a month I had gone from displaying unexplained symptoms to the first of eight rounds of chemo. My oncologist's reasoning behind hitting a particularly aggressive cancer with similar force was simple but effective: "I don't want to have to treat this again a few years down the line," he said.

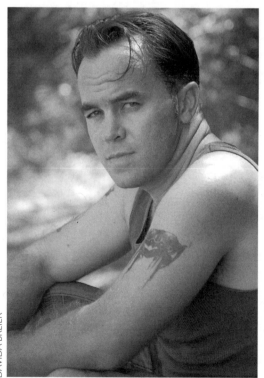

DAVIDA BREIER

Guides to the Planet

William Patrick Tandy was diagnosed with Stage II-B non-Hodgkin's lymphoma in March 2007 and quickly learned that chemotherapy is not nearly as fun as they make it look on television. Knock on wood, six months of R-CHOP did the trick. Since 2001 his Eight-Stone Press imprint (www.eightstonepress.com) has published the award-winning *Smile, Hon, You're in Baltimore!* series to popular and critical fanfare.

> All the doctors involved
> handled my case with
> professionalism and empathy.

> Ask about every possible
> fertility option before your
> treatment starts. If your chemo
> needed to begin yesterday—
> if it did begin yesterday—ask
> anyway. If you're twenty-three
> and you think you'll ever want
> kids, *ask anyway!*

{ Don't freak out! (OK, freak out for five minutes, then get a grip. You're allowed to do this periodically, BTW.) }

Chapter Two

Getting Your C-Legs

Holy. Shit. It's all different now. Everything.
— MEMYSELFEYE

I was chatting with a friend about becoming a pirate. He commented on how I would probably develop scurvy. He then retracted his statement on the grounds that the last time he predicted I would get a disease, brain cancer, it actually came true.

— RYAN JARTA

The bad news is out. Cancer. You or someone you're close to has it. That sucks. Now we must pile on some more bad news: You have to get in front of this freight train but not let it bulldoze you. You have to get organized, and you have to stay that way. That's right. Amid all this mania and frustration, helplessness and fear, amid your life getting minced in a blender and served in tiny cups to a bunch of white-coated people you didn't know a month ago, you have to keep it real and prepare to be your own advocate/soldier/secretary.

Don't freak out! (OK, freak out for five minutes, then get a grip. You're allowed to do this periodically, BTW.) This chapter helps you take control of the situation and maintain the upper hand. You'll learn how to navigate your insurance situation (or lack of one) and what legal legs you have to stand on. You'll also receive a little education about the various intimidatingly named tests, machines, and devices you're about to encounter, so you'll be knowledgeable about what's coming down the pike as you start exploring the Planet via your treatment regimen.

Finding out you have cancer is overwhelming and frightening and surprising and crappy, yes; but, that crappiness notwithstanding, you don't want to enter your treatment as a hapless pinball, getting bounced around between hospital and home without knowing what's going on and without any say as to what's happening to you. So read up; let's go!

Things and People That Steer Your Treatment

To diagnose your cancer and, subsequently, to monitor it, your oncologist(s) will choose from a mind-boggling array of tests and scans. Below you'll find some of the main types of scans and tests for easy reference, complete with definitions and some stories to illustrate their upsides and downsides. And, occasionally, backsides. After that we include a list of people who will assist with the practical issues that accompany cancer treatment.

Pencils ready? Game on!

Everything Starts with a Pathology Report

The pathologist is the most important person you'll (probably) never meet. Although your oncologist is responsible for your final diagnosis after reviewing all the necessary tests, scans, and biopsies, the pathology report from the person in the back hunched over a microscope is a critical piece of the puzzle.

Have your doctor go over the pathology report with you. Even before you do that, though, make sure the report is yours! Your name and other identifying info, such as your birth date, will be on it. Also, make sure that your pathologist is board-certified. If you have a rare diagnosis, it's especially worth it to have slides and tissue samples reviewed by an expert pathologist at a cancer center to confirm or correct the diagnosis.

The pathology report documents, where applicable, both what a surgeon noted about your tumor's appearance during your biopsy—what was visible to the naked eye—and the conclusions of the pathologist who examined the tissue samples under a microscope.

In addition to proposing a diagnosis, the pathology report includes information about the characteristics of the tumor such as "stage" and "grade," meaning: how big the tumor is, whether and how much the cancer has spread, and how aggressive the particular type of cancer is.

Get a copy of the report for your own records. Ask questions and take notes. Make sure that your doc explains any unfamiliar terms to you. That way, instead of walking out of there hearing only the word "cancer" ringing in your ears, you'll have more information about just what you're up against.

Demystifying the Complete Blood Count Test (CBC)

You'll be giving blood a lot during treatment, as the levels of your red and white blood cells and platelets are one of the standard ways to measure your treatment's progress. Ranges vary according to factors such as patient age, gender, and test method, so it's important to talk to your doctor to find out exactly what is normal for you. As you read below, keep in mind that the highs and lows of the numbers don't mean much clinically unless they're really, really high or really, really low, and the art of treating cancer is, based on those highs and lows, figuring out when to act, and how. Understandably, each doctor will do this a little differently.

The CBC will become the marker that dictates the progress (or slow-gress, or, in some cases, no-gress) of your days and weeks in cancer treatment, as low counts may cause your doctor to postpone treatment until your counts recover. So when the doctor pulls out this hieroglyphic printout and starts going over it with you, it makes sense for you to know what the hell it means. Or at least what the important parts of it are, and what they mean. Here we present a primer for reading your own blood test. Bring on the CBC!

IMPORTANT TERMS

WBC: White blood cells are your immune system's key players in the fight against infection. The WBC is a count of the actual number of WBCs per volume of blood. A normal WBC count varies from person to person, and you should confirm with your doc what's normal for you, but generally a level of 4,500 to 10,000 white blood cells per microliter (mcL) is considered normal.

More is not always better, though: Leukemia patients go wildly out of range on the upper end of WBCs, crowding out the red blood cells and platelets.

Depending on your treatment, you may receive medicine, sometimes called "growth factors," to help boost your white count or red count. Often while recovering from chemotherapy, your white count may be high—usually this is something your doctors just keep an eye on. (Sometimes the white count can be high due to stress, steroids, or infection.)

Differential: Shown as a percentage, the differential measures the five types of WBCs present in the blood, each of which has a different role in protecting us from infection. The five types are neutrophils (aka segs, PMNs, polys, grans), lymphocytes, monocytes, eosinophils, and basophils.

The neutrophils are the front-line soldiers (see ANC below) and make up about 60 percent of the total WBC number. The lymphocytes, second-line fighters, make up about 25 percent.

Monocytes, basophils, and eosinophils make up the rest of the white blood cell count and usually have relatively low percentages except in certain cases, such as specific leukemias or allergic responses. Your doc isn't quite as concerned about these guys. File this one under "Man, my doc will think I'm a genius if I know . . . ": Your monocytes recover faster than your neutrophils, so your differential might show the percentage of monocytes as abnormally high after chemotherapy before your neutrophils recover to normal levels.

ANC: Absolute neutrophil count. Neutrophils are the white blood cells required to fight bacterial infection. Your oncologist will observe this reading closely. If your ANC is below 1,000, you are probably *neutropenic,* which means that you are particularly susceptible to infections. A fever in a patient with neutropenia requires prompt antibiotic therapy, often in the hospital. If you have a fever with a low ANC, even a small infection can become a big deal, so if you have a fever and your counts are low, call your doctor, no questions.

RBC: Red blood cells. If you're feeling sluggish and tired, which is common in treatment, expect a low RBC number. Red blood cells are the oxygen transporters in your blood and thus are a good indicator of your energy level. The RBC is a count of the actual number of red blood cells per volume of blood. Again, what's normal varies from person to person, but generally for men, 4.7 million to 6.1 million cells per microliter (cells/mcL) is considered normal. For women it's 4.2 million to 5.4 million cells/mcL.

Hb or Hgb: Hemoglobin. This measures the amount of oxygen-carrying protein in the blood. An Hb less than 10 generally means that you have symptomatic anemia, which can cause fatigue, breathlessness, or poor exercise tolerance. Your doctor might consider a shot such as Procrit or Aranesp to raise the blood count.

Hct: Hematocrit, shown as a percentage indicating the amount of space that RBCs take up in the blood. It's usually three times the hemoglobin. It's a calculated number, however, so it's not always exact. Most doctors usually use either hemoglobin or hematocrit to determine when an intervention—a transfusion or a shot, not a meeting with a tight circle of concerned relatives—is needed. If the hemoglobin is less than around 7 and the hematocrit less than around 20, your doctor might consider a transfusion. This is very doctor-dependent and has a fair amount to do with how you're doing clinically. That is, if you're showing no symptoms, your doc might decide not to transfuse.

Plts: Platelets, the key player in blood clotting. This is a count of the actual number of platelets in a given volume of blood. Normal

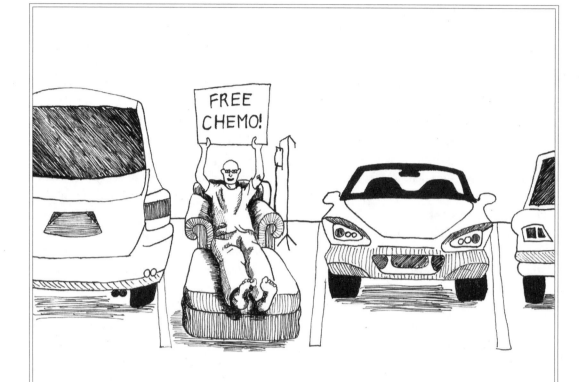

Top 10 Ways to Disrupt the Waiting Room

10. Ask everyone around you to do things "STAT."

9. Offer free prostate exams.

8. Ask everyone nervously for a spare catheter.

7. Pop a disc in the DVD player of you in an avocado-eating contest.

6. Supplement bland waiting room periodicals with nurse-fetish pornography.

5. Give your best rendition of that dance-floor classic: The Naked Raptor.

4. Hold up a sign that reads, "Free chemo in the parking lot."

3. Initiate a spelling bee. Be unflinchingly cruel with errors.

2. Leaf through every magazine in the room, shake hands with everyone else, and then say loudly, "Jesus, this flesh-eating scabies itches like a mother."

1. Repeatedly refer to the doctor you're waiting to see as "The Trembling Butcher."

falls between 130,000 and 350,000/mcL, which your doctor will describe simply as "130–350." A normal platelet count can be knocked out of whack by chemotherapy (which makes it drop). Cancer can make the platelet count too high (this is called an "acute phase reactant," a term that sounds cribbed from *Star Trek*). Time or transfusions will bring the count back up after chemotherapy; if the count is too high, treatment will usually bring it down to normal levels.

Everything You (N)ever Wanted to Know About Scans

There are many types of scans that image your insides from different angles. It's good to know the (sometimes slight) differences among the various scans you'll undergo.

X-ray: An oldie but a goodie. X-rays use electromagnetic radiation to produce an image of some part of your body. X-rays aren't as sophisticated (or as expensive!) as many of the newer types of tests, but they can still be useful for finding and monitoring some types of tumors.

CT or CAT Scan: Stands for "computed tomography." A CT scanner looks like a big doughnut. It builds a 3-D picture of your insides using a series of X-rays taken from different angles. To be scanned, you might first have to drink barium, get a barium enema, or be injected with a contrast dye that increases the visual difference between normal and abnormal tissue. Or all of the above. Then you lie on a table that goes back and forth through the middle hole of the doughnut. The scanner rotates around you inside the doughnut, whirring and clicking. CT scans generally aren't painful, although if your scan takes an hour or more, it can be hard to stay still, and you may have to

hold your breath at certain points, depending on what is being scanned. Oh, and barium is disgusting. (See "What It's Really Like to . . . Get a CT Scan" later in this chapter.)

MRI: Stands for "magnetic resonance imaging." An MRI does *not* use radiation—instead, it uses magnetic fields to create a detailed cross section of the area being scanned, including soft tissue and internal organs. Because MRIs use ultra-strong magnets, you need to give full disclosure of all metal implants in your body—don't forget any random piercings—before having an MRI. (Or else the generally painless MRI may become *very* painful.)

Depending on the area being scanned, you may or may not have an injection of a contrast dye. Then you lie down on a table that slides into the MRI, which resembles a tube or tunnel—how far in you go depends on the area being scanned. (If you're claustrophobic, you may want to request a sedative beforehand or see if an Open MRI—which has more space around the body—is an option for you.) While the machine is scanning, you'll hear a series of loud (and we mean loud) knocks. These knocking sounds are the gradient coils in the machine vibrating—gradient coils, which are pretty much wire encased in plastic, do this because of the rapid rate at which the electric current passing through the wire is switched off and on (every few milliseconds). Each knocking sound indicates that it is creating a different view of your insides. You'll need to remain still during scanning, which is done in a series with short breaks in between and may last up to 90 minutes.

Ultrasound: It's not just for pregnancies anymore! Ultrasounds create pictures of your internal organs using high-frequency sound

---

Criteria for MRI Playlists

1. **Need to be around an hour long.**

2. **Should be loud enough to drown out the jackhammer noises.**

3. **Upbeat tempo, but not so toe-tappy that the techs have to do the scan again!**

---

waves. (Believe it or not, tumors bounce back sound waves differently from normal tissue.) The equipment includes a computer, a video screen, and a small handheld device called a "transducer." Ultrasounds are usually painless and last twenty minutes to an hour.

While you are lying on the exam table, generally on your back or side, the technician spreads a water-soluble gel on your skin over the area to be scanned. (If you're lucky, they'll use gel warmers, because that stuff can be *cold*.) The technician places the transducer against your skin and moves it around, periodically capturing the images produced on the computer for a radiologist to review.

PET scan: Stands for "positron emission tomography." A PET scan creates an image of radioactive activity in your body—not that cancer is radioactive. The test involves injecting a small amount of radioactive sugar molecules. Because cancer cells absorb sugar faster than regular cells, cancerous hot spots show up brightly on a PET scan. For a PET scan you'll need to be NPO (*Nil per os*, a Latin phrase meaning "nothing by mouth." Don't eat or drink anything for four to six hours) and have no sugar before the procedure.

After the initial injection, you'll lie quietly for thirty to ninety minutes to give the contrast time to reach the body parts being scanned; then you'll be taken to the scanner, which, like a CT machine, resembles a large doughnut. (In fact, it is not uncommon to have a combination PET/CT scan.) You'll need to lie very still on the exam table, which will slide back and forth through the hole in the middle of the scanner over the next thirty to sixty minutes. PET scans are generally painless.

Bone scan: This test involves injecting a radioactive tracer into the body. The tracer will be picked up in the bones and reveal any damage, whether from cancer or another cause. After the initial injection, you'll have to wait one to four hours for the tracer to spread throughout your bones. (Drink lots of water during this period to make sure you pee out tracer that's going places besides your bones, like your kidneys or bladder.) For the scan, you'll lie on an exam table while a camera passes over and/or around your body, creating a lovely visual of your skeleton. A bone scan takes thirty to sixty minutes and is not painful, although you'll have to lie still the whole time.

A great resource for more information on various tests and scans is in the "Treatments, Tests, and Procedures" section of Cancer.net, the patient-focused Web site developed by the American Society of Clinical Oncology.

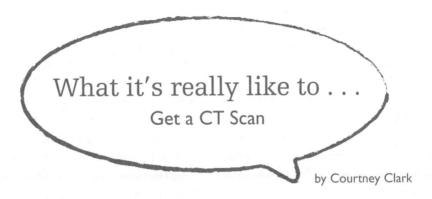

What it's really like to . . .
Get a CT Scan

by Courtney Clark

Getting a CT scan is like water torture: There's no moment where you've reached a pinnacle of pain. Instead, the whole process is a series of indignities and discomforts heaped upon you for a few ugly hours. At University of Texas M.D. Anderson Cancer Center in Houston, they perform triple-contrast CT scanning for better viewing. Triple-contrast is a pleasant way of saying you're going to be drinking disgusting barium, have a barium enema shoved up your behind, and have radioactive iodine injected into your veins.

For me, the first injustice was not being able to eat for hours beforehand. As far as I'm concerned, withhold food and anyone deserves to be cranky. When you finally get to put something in your stomach, though, it isn't what you'd want. Barium is a thick, chalky substance that People Who Never Had Cancer have tried to disguise with flavors like "berry," "apple," "pina colada," and "banana." The bad news is you have to drink it all. The good news is you have half an hour to do so. The bad news is it'll still be hard to finish.

While you are drinking, enjoy the company of the other cancer patients in the waiting room, all drinking the same barium. Many of them have had CT procedures before, and you can get a rousing discussion going on liquid barium strategy and which flavors are better. Just wait. You have to drink three glasses of the stuff, so you'll get chances to experiment.

After the first two glasses, your stomach will start to feel like lead. When you start the third glass, a tech will call you back into the radiology rooms and start getting you prepped. If you don't have a port, they'll put an IV in your vein for the iodine and hopefully wrap you up in a blanket to wait and finish your last frosty cold barium beverage.

At this point during my first CT scan, a very kindly (and by that I mean attractive and young) male nurse pulled me aside to tell me that the iodine injection makes you feel as though you are wetting yourself. He reminded me not to freak out and get up from the table, because you aren't actually peeing on yourself, but it feels like it.

Iodine allergies are swift and problematic, so during your first CT scan they'll be watching you closely to make sure you don't have a reaction. If you have a reaction—difficulty breathing or swelling of your tongue or throat—you'll know it immediately and so will the techs, and they'll rush in with an injection. Iodine allergies can also develop with repeated exposure, so some patients with long cancer histories can't have iodine anymore.

At this point the barium is weighing heavily in your stomach, you are freaking out about peeing yourself, and they escort you into the room with the

CT scan. The machine is shaped like a doughnut, and you lie on a table that slides back and forth through the doughnut. Then the tech comes in and asks you to roll on one side and lower your scrub pants. Your barium enema begins, and the tech hooks you up to the iodine. As she pushes the iodine and leaves the room, you feel like you have to pee. But the weirdest part of the iodine experience is the intense heat and not-totally-unenjoyable tingly feeling straight down the center of your face and torso.

The iodine sensations evaporate, and you start rolling back and forth through the doughnut while either the machine-robot voice or the tech tells you when to breathe and when to hold your breath. The scanning usually takes between five and thirty minutes, and by that time you are embarrassingly aware that the barium enema wasn't the only pain in the ass today brought.

Once the iodine drip is removed, the only thing on your mind should be eating real food to replace the taste of barium. I craved savory, salty, meaty foods after my scans—anything that was the complete opposite of the thick, sweet goo. You feel bloated and gassy afterward for about half a day, but at least you made it through the day without peeing on yourself.

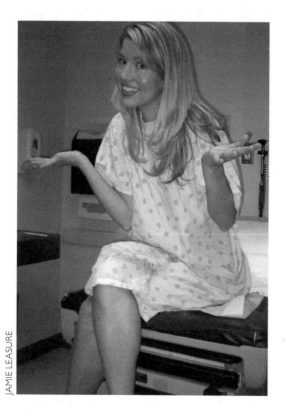

JAMIE LEASURE

Guides to the Planet

Courtney Clark, a melanoma survivor, has served as director of development and marketing for Planet Cancer and currently runs Austin Involved, a young professional volunteer group. She credits her surgeon, Dr. Merrick Ross, and a whacked-out sense of humor for saving her life. Spending time as the only young adult in the M.D. Anderson waiting room earned her a new respect for the families of cancer fighters, as well as lots of requests for dates with people's grandchildren. When Courtney isn't rescuing her friends from tanning beds, she rescues puppies from shelters and leftover pasta from other people's plates. Courtney hates hearing this: "Skin cancer isn't really cancer." She hopes that by handling their disease with grace and humor, young adults with cancer will pave the way for their peers, who'll likely be where we are someday.

Barium . . . Yum, yum! (Not.)

Depending on what's being examined, you might have to down a totally disgusting barium drink before your CT scan. Barium absorbs X-rays, so it helps highlight irregularities anywhere in the drink's path—the pharynx, esophagus, and on down. If you have taste buds and a soul, you will hate the barium drink. It looks a little like grade-school glue cut with water. A CT scan takes less than an hour, usually; getting over the barium drink takes much, much longer. Like forever. Though the barium drink supposedly is not to be mixed with anything, some sympathetic doctors and nurses have been known to allow dilution with clear diet sodas (sugar can botch the scan). If you don't have such liberal staff on your Planet, go old school and chug it. Make sure you bring a toothbrush to get the taste out of your mouth as quickly as possible.

{ Yes I Want Morphine, Buddy! }

by Jen Singer

This essay originally appeared on GoodHousekeeping.com.

It would have been funny even if I wasn't on morphine at the time. Funny in that twisted way that comes to cancer patients like me and the families who love them and understand they really need a good laugh at the oddest times. The doctor, however, was not amused, and yet, he started it.

I was lying facedown on my hospital bed for a bone marrow test. I'll save the squeamish from the gory details. Just know that it hurt and it was harrowing. Midway through the procedure, the doctor asked me, "Have you ever had morphine?" I answered through gritted teeth, "Yup." He added, "Did you tolerate it well?" I forced, "Yup." He asked, "Would you like some now?"

Would I like some morphine now? In the middle of a bone marrow test? I would indeed like some now, and perhaps a glass of water if it's not too much trouble. YES, I WANT MORPHINE, BUDDY! Why he didn't ask me that before he started extracting a sample of my bone, I don't know. But some people are better hosts than others, I suppose.

As soon he gave me the morphine and continued the procedure, his phone rang. What kind of ring tone does an oncologist program into his phone? Simon and Garfunkel's "Bridge Over Troubled Water," maybe? A simple, old-fashioned phone ring, perhaps? Or just program it to vibrate?

No, in the middle of my bone marrow test—to see if the cancer had spread (and it hadn't)—my doctor's cell phone played "Bohemian Rhapsody" by Queen. You know the song: "I see a little silhouetto of a man. Scaramouche, Scaramouche, will you do the fandango? Thunderbolt and lightning—very, very frightening, me."

Which is why, in the middle of my bone marrow test (and after the morphine kicked in), I began to sing, "Galileo! Galileo! Galileo! Galileo! Galileo Figaro! Magnifico—But I'm just a poor boy and nobody loves me."

And then my husband chimed in, "He's just a poor boy from a poor family. Spare him his life from this monstrosity."

When the phone stopped playing Queen and my husband and I finished our duet, the doctor sighed in resignation and said, "You're going to write about me, aren't you?"

Scaramouche, Doc. Scaramouche. But hey, at least you didn't answer the phone.

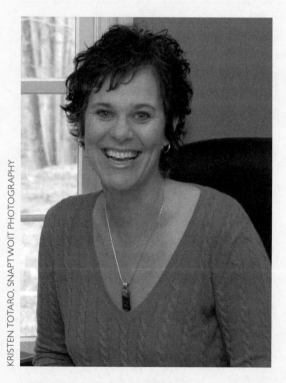

KRISTEN TOTARO, SNAPTWOIT PHOTOGRAPHY

Guides to the Planet

Jen Singer was diagnosed with aggressive B-cell non-Hodgkin's lymphoma at age forty. Her doctor originally staged her cancer at III, but she negotiated him down to a II. "OK," she writes, "so maybe the tumor the size of a softball in my lung technically hung a little bit below my diaphragm, thus making it Stage III. But if he didn't give me what I wanted, I just might have started a strike outside his office. And nobody wants to see a bald woman carrying a sign and shouting. Not even in New York City." Her cancer is now in remission. She wrote parts of her book *You're a Good Mom (and Your Kids Aren't So Bad Either)* while staying on the oncology floor in the hospital. The creator of the award-winning MommaSaid.net and the author of the *Stop Second-Guessing Yourself* guides to parenting, Jen is the mom of two boys who talk to her through the bathroom door.

Ultrasound
by Anna Peled

Like the hero of a low-budget action film
I am clinging desperately
To his silences
And reaching to be rescued
By his words.
Like a carnival fortune teller
I am peering into his eyes
For any reflection
Of what he is seeing.
I am reading my future
In each minute expression
On his young, kind face.
I don't want to talk about school.
I want to talk about why the probe
Is lingering so long on that one spot
On the lower right side of my abdomen.
Pushing and prodding.
Searching and sliding.
You can forget that good health is a gift
Until you are lying in a cold room
Trying to focus only on the mother tiger
    and her baby
In the cheap metal frame.

Fun with Catheters

I lost my port two times, and my veins were not doing well. I knew I was in for a five- to six-hour session of chemo intravenously. The nurse asked why I was looking "a little green," and I told her I was nervous about the corrosive chemicals that would be going into my very sore hand, and that I had a fear of getting "burned." Her words—

I kid you not—"Well, it's not like a port makes you safe. I once saw a man with a Hickman [a type of external port] lose half his chest wall before we knew it was leaking!" Talk about reassurance.

—KayCee

Catheters, or venous access devices (VADs), are used to deliver drugs, nutrients, blood, platelets, and/or fluids directly into a main vein in the body; going the other direction, they are used as ready access points for drawing blood. Catheters are great: They're like a superhighway for whatever you're putting in your body. And by eliminating the constant search for a "good" vein, they save the veins in your hands and arms from constant poking, prodding, irritation, and potential collapse.

There are two kinds of catheters:

Internal catheters are located completely under the skin. When you're not hooked up to an IV, an internal catheter is not visible, except possibly as a lump underneath your skin or . . . oh, wait, that big ol' scar from the surgical insertion. It's accessed through the skin using a special angled needle. (Yes, you want nurses with good aim.)

External catheters are also surgically implanted and anchored onto a large internal vein, but with tubes extending through the skin for easy access. Gives a whole new meaning to "letting it all hang out." Generally, external catheters are more of a bother than internal ones, in that they require bandage changes every other day and flushes every day. Internal catheters only need to be flushed once a month and after use; additionally, you can swim, bathe, etc., with them much more easily than with external catheters.

A doctor takes several factors into consideration when deciding what type of catheter to use, including:

- Patient's age and size

- Length of time the catheter will be in place

- Purpose of the catheter (For example, if there is a strong likelihood of needing TPN, you may get a triple lumen catheter with three tubes hanging out. For the overachievers.)

- Patient's previous history with catheters

- Condition of the blood vessels

- Special needs of the patient

- Personal preference

Types of External Catheters
- **Hickman:** Placed in the chest during out-patient surgery and tunneled under the skin into a central blood vessel, with several tubes protruding outside the skin. Can remain in place for extended periods.

TPN stands for "total parenteral nutrition," yummy nutritional formulas that you can receive through your catheter when you can't get food down. Contains tasty things like salts, glucose, amino acids, lipids, and vitamins.

- **Broviac:** The Hickman's smaller cousin. No reason why it sounds like a personified main-frame computer from an eighties movie.

- **Groshong:** Similar to Hickman and Broviac, but with a different tip. Probably named after the sinister German operator of the aforementioned mainframe.

- **PICC (Peripherally Inserted Central Catheter) Line:** A long plastic catheter inserted into an arm vein. PICC lines are more temporary than Hickman ports and port-a-caths because they can inhibit movement, but they can still last months with proper insertion and maintenance.

Types of Internal Catheters
- **Port-a-cath:** Also known as a port, infuse-a-port, or mediport. A blob of self-sealing sili-cone set in a titanium or plastic housing with one or two lumens (openings) leading into a silicone catheter threaded into the vein. It kind of looks like Mickey Mouse ears. Ports are surgically implanted, typically below the clavicle (Planet Cancer can introduce you to some cool words; "subclavian" is one), but they can also be implanted near the rib cage. They are designed to sustain five hundred to two thousand punctures.

- **PASport:** More recent to the catheter world and yet to be widely favored by doctors, PAS-ports are smaller than port-a-caths and can be inserted in the upper arm instead of the chest. A welcome advance for those who favor low-cut necklines.

{ Point People as You Navigate the Planet }

by Stacia Wagner
Director of Survivor Programs,
Children's Brain Tumor Foundation

Social Worker

Each oncology team should have an oncology social worker, who should be someone you can talk to about concrete needs as well as emotional needs. If you have not met one, ask your doc to make the introduction. This person should have special training on the ins and outs of services like insurance, SSI/SSDI, Medicaid, employment issues, and resources. For specific services, you may need to be assertive and ask for assistance.

Here are some things you should be able to go to your social worker for:

- What qualifies a person for SSI/SSDI (see "What Is Medicaid?" later in the chapter), and how do you apply for it? (Tip: Ask the social worker if he or she has a contact at the SSI office who can speed up the application process.) Social workers can also assist with completing the application.

- How to talk to your employer about what you need, including extended time off. What accommodations can you ask for at work and what is not realistic? (See "A Brief Tidbit about Your Workplace" later in the chapter.)

- How do you explain your résumé when you go back to looking for work and there is a gap?

If the social worker does not know, ask her about cancer-related employment resources. (See "Going Back to Work" in chapter 7.) If your social worker is not familiar with these, try the local college career center.

- Health insurance can provide lots of challenges. Your social worker is one of the many people who can assist you with resources that might help with uncovered drugs and services, the ins and outs of Medicaid, finding insurance coverage, and whom to talk to about specific bills. (See "Insurance Alphabet Soup" later in the chapter.)

- Communicating, mediating, and coordinating with the rest of the medical team. The social worker can arrange for team meetings to assist in understanding any medical questions or concerns you have. If you want her to act as your representative in getting questions answered, she can do that as well.

- Transportation/lodging and any day-to-day needs you have. Social workers can assist you with resources for all of the practical issues that come along with a cancer diagnosis. They can be really great go-to people. If there's no resource for your needs, the social worker should have access to other social workers who may be able to come up with answers.

- If you are going to need assistance when you go home (someone to stay with you, home "improvements," etc.), the social worker can link you to the resources you need.

Hospital Patient Advocate/ Representative

This person should be able to act as your spokesperson. If for some reason the hospital does not have patient advocates or you want an extra one, you may want to ask someone you are comfortable with or who you know is smart and assertive to fill the role. Some things this person should be able to do:

- Navigate what is going on. In addition to the medical team, the advocate should be able to explain all of the medical jargon, clinical trials, informed consents, tests, procedures, and treatment choices. If the advocate doesn't know the answers, he or she will ask the questions and help you get them.

- Planning and scheduling. If you want your advocate to assist you with scheduling appointments or tracking medications, let him or her know. Think about what type of scheduling works best for you. Do you want appointments on the same day or spread out? How much information do you want to share with your advocate? Do you want the person to come with you to appointments? If not, how will the advocate get an update? Make sure you let your docs know who your advocate is, what the person is going to do for you, and his or her contact information.

- Records-keeper. Your advocate can keep written documentation of your schedule, your treatment, your reactions to treatment, and the answers to your questions.

- Spokesperson. Your advocate can be your spokesperson with both the medical team and your friends and family. The situation may change, but if there are times you want the advocate to let people know what is going on, he or she should be able to fill that role.

Hospital Finance Department Representative

It is helpful if you can meet with a representative from the finance department as soon as possible. This person can help you understand:

- What your insurance will cover and what percentage of services will be covered

- When you will and when you won't need pre-authorization for services

- Financial assistance provided by the hospital and how to negotiate what you need to pay

In order to eliminate spending countless hours on the phone with your insurance company, you can ask the representative to talk to your insurance company about policy issues. You can also have the representative review and explain your bills.

These services are in most patient financial representatives' job descriptions, but the quality and expertise vary from hospital to hospital and person to person. You may have better luck working directly with your health insurance representative (see below). However, the hospital representative will know the hospital billing, prescription, and authorization system better than anyone else.

Health Insurance Representative

This person can be a lifesaver. Key to getting good service is calling the representative number listed on your health insurance card. You will need to know your policy/group and/or member number. Ask the representative some basic questions about your policy. (What percentage of drugs is covered? Do I need to ask for generic when possible? How do I get a referral for out-of-network services?) If this person is helpful and courteous, keep his or her name. It helps to have one contact person as she or he will be familiar with your case and you will not have to repeat yourself.

This person will be able to answer questions on:

- Co-pays
- Premiums
- Lifetime maximum
- Going out-of-network
- Second opinions
- Clinical trial coverage
- Complementary/alternative medicine coverage
- Coverage for services such as at-home nursing and equipment
- Exclusions
- Out-of-pocket expenses
- Co-insurance

Hey Left Brain:

Some Jobs for You

You have no idea what being organized will do for you on Planet Cancer. It makes you a formidable force in your own treatment: You can take on your insurance company with confidence and bust out treatment records if a doctor has a question. Being organized also gives you confidence about your own recent medical history, which, let's face it, you wouldn't remember jack about if you weren't keeping good notes and records (see "Chemo Brain" in chapter 4). Six months down the road (and much later), you'll be happy if you've kept copious records—in addition to ably substituting for your memory, it can give you a relieving feeling of control.

Three main areas will require some organizational attention:

1. **Treatment:** Your doctors' visits, hospitalizations, treatment plan, tests, scans, and various other details related to your medical care.

2. **Medication:** Worth a good system, especially for transplant patients and others with a truckload of prescriptions. The last thing you want

> The last thing you want is for your occasional fogginess of the brain to result in a dangerous medication mix-up.

is for your occasional fogginess of the brain to result in a dangerous medication mix-up.

3. **Financials:** Everything related to insurance companies or public assistance. What you're billed for, what you've paid for, and what someone else has paid for.

It's not just about getting and staying organized, however; it's also about taking care of some imperative paperwork—your advance directives. Read on for your crash course in Cancer Organization 101.

Keeping Track of Treatments

There are a number of different notebooks and systems out there designed to help cancer patients going through treatment. You can explore and find one that works for you or make up your own. Maybe you're a paper person; maybe you swear by your PDA. But no matter what the format, all systems should cover several key elements in order to be effective.

1. The calendar.

Obviously, this is the place to set down all your doctor's appointments, but it can also serve as sort of a medical diary. By that, we mean that you can keep track of other things, such as:

- When you ran a fever.

- When you threw up all night.

- What time you took that last Percocet so you know when you can take the next one.

- When you refilled your prescription.

> **Tip:** When talking to anyone at any agency, take note of the person's name, the time, what was said, etc., in addition to asking for direct lines, so that referencing the conversation to supervisors, or citing info to others, is easily managed. If you want to take the lazy/convenient route, just record the conversation.

- What time your appointment was scheduled vs. when it actually started. If your doctor is always an hour late, why not start calling ahead to check so you can gauge your own arrival accordingly?

- When you started and ended shots to boost your white or red blood cell count and what your counts were before and after.

This way, you can go back and skim through to see the trends in your treatment and note the ups and downs and the recovery time. It makes it easier to get through the downs if you can look back and realize that, eventually, you came back up! If you're the electronic type, you can also set alarms for when you need to take meds. (See "Managing Your Meds" later in the chapter.)

2. Test results and records.

Every time you have a test or a scan—CBC, CT scan, whatevs—get a copy of the report and file it here. This is for your own reference and also to make sure that, as you quarterback your medical team, all members have access to the same information. So when Doc #1 asks you a question about the last CT scan that Doc #4 ordered, you have the date, time, and results on hand. Keep notes on discussions about any tests attached to the relevant test results. Be sure to note the date of any such discussion, who was included in the conversation, and the outcome or any action items.

3. Notes on treatment and communications with your health-care team.

How many times have you walked out of a doctor's office and thirty minutes later you can't recount exactly what was said? That's why you need a notebook in which either you, a friend, or a family member can take notes, both for your own reference and, again, to relay accurate information to the various members of your team.

Keep that sucker close at hand to record not only the scheduled conversations but the questions that pop into your head at 3 a.m. or when you're in line at the grocery store. Write them down so you'll have them ready for your next call or appointment.

This is also a good place to make note of things you want to remember—things that help or hurt; for example, if you found that a particular type of tea helped settle your stomach in the hospital or that you like button-front shirts best when you're hooked up to an IV, write it down on a hospital checklist of things to remember for the next time you check in.

4. Contact information for every medical professional you see.

Get some of those plastic pages with inserts for business cards, and every time you see a new health-care professional, grab his or her card. Also, keep multiple photocopies of a contact list that you've typed up as a computer document and keep it updated when you add new docs. Be sure to include the dates you saw them. It will save you adding "writer's cramp" or "carpal tunnel syndrome" to your list of diagnoses when you have to fill out medical forms that ask what doctors you've seen, when, and why. (In those teeny-tiny spaces too! The nerve.) Just hand them your printed list and be done with it.

Super Sneaky Tip: When you're in the hospital or clinic, keep an eye out for posted lists of the phone/pager numbers for various members of your medical team. They leave them there for each other, but if they haven't given them to you already, store them in your phone in case you need them. For example, if the nurse won't call you back to answer a question, you can go straight to your doc.

{ Mastering Your Meds }

by JT Burns

You know how most people set an alarm to wake themselves up in the mornings? Well, see, I'm in my first one hundred days post-transplant and I don't have a life to get to in the mornings, so instead I set my iPhone alarms for med times so I won't forget to take anything.

When you're taking like a hundred different things, it's easy to lose track. To make sure that I don't take anything twice or forget to take something, I have a big chart of what I have to take and when to take it. I just go down the line and check off when I take it. Once I'm done with a certain med, I'll move it from the main pile to another "station" to get it out of my way and so I won't have to worry about it anymore. I mark the tops of all the bottles with a different colored marker. For example, green means that I have to take it more than once a day. Orange means I take it only once, in the morning. My favorites are the blue markings: Those are the "as needed" meds like Ativan, Dilaudid. Mmmmmmm. Anyway, the only purpose those markings serve are to have the meds be easily identifiable. I hate more than anything having to read all the labels on all the bottles to find what I need. If I'm looking for a pain med, I know right off the bat to look at the blue markings. At one point, I had them organized by color and then in alphabetical order within the color, but I got too lazy to keep it that way.

I'm just the kind of guy who needs to take his meds from the containers. If I put them in bags or try the pillbox thing, I get nervous because some of them I take at different times and I just always need to make sure I know what I'm taking and when.

Besides, there's no pillbox big enough for what I need to take. If I tried to stuff my pills into the box labeled "Monday," I could only fit, like, two. So what do I do with the other million?

Financial and Legal Concerns

When it comes to being organized, this is where the rubber meets the road. When you're dealing with medical bills, there are just a couple of categories of paper to be pushed, but keeping them organized and cross-referenced makes all the difference in the world.

The Bill: This is from the provider, i.e., the licensed professional (physician, radiologist, oncologist, etc.) or institution (hospital, clinic, skilled nursing facility, etc.) that provided the service. It should be organized by Date of Service (DOS) and should itemize whatever you had done, how much it cost, any discounts given or payments made, and the remaining balance to be paid by you. If it's not itemized, ask for an itemized bill. And keep in mind that it can take a couple of bills to get to the correct final tally, especially if your insurance company processes things slowly. So never pay it right off the bat!

Also, when you see medical professionals in the hospital—anesthesiologists, radiologists, oncologists—know that it's not all a package deal for billing purposes and they each might have separate charges. So, for example, you might receive separate bills from the surgeon, the hospital, and the anesthesiologist for one surgical procedure.

The Explanation of Benefits (EOB): This is from the insurer. It should be organized by DOS also and should reflect who provided the service, how much was charged, how much the insurance company will cover, how much it will pay, how much is applied to any deductible, and—at the end of all that—how much you owe. The EOB is not a bill. It just shows how much your insurance company will pay on each line item of the provider's invoice. When you compare the EOB to the actual bill, the two documents should reflect the same final total of money you owe. Or don't.

Everyone has a preference for how to manage the mountains of paper in these two categories, but if you're just getting started, here's a suggestion for setting up your process.

Get an accordion folder for documents received in a calendar year and create four files:

1. **Bills for which you have not received an EOB yet.** Organize them by DOS.

2. **EOBs for which you have not received a bill yet.** It can happen.

3. **Settled bills.** When you or your insurer pays off a bill, write the date of payment and (if you paid) how you paid—check number or credit card used. Staple the bills (you might have several months' worth) and EOBs together and file here. Group bills by provider and organize by DOS for easy reference.

4. **Matched-up bills and EOBs that are not closed out.** This is the stack of bills that are being disputed, negotiated, paid off on a payment plan, or otherwise have details that still need to be finalized.

The thing about medical bills is that they can require a lot of back-and-forth between you, the provider, and the insurer before they get paid off. So get ready to spend a lot of time on the phone and take a lot of notes. It's easiest to just take notes directly on the bill or EOB—you can attach extra pages if necessary.

With every call you make, take the following information:

- Date and time of call

- Name of the person you are speaking with and that person's direct phone number

- What was discussed and the outcome of the conversation

- If there is any follow-up or callback required—and put it on your calendar

This should help you keep documents at hand, easy to find and ready to act on. When you start a new calendar year, get a new accordion folder so that you can start fresh, along with your deductible!

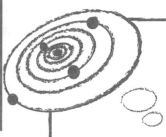

Dispatches
from the Planet

My family members are the most unorganized, unable to remember anything a doctor says, don't want to ask questions, don't rock the boat people in the world. I have no shame and would ask a doctor any question at any time. If they did not have an answer, I politely asked who did.

We were managing multiple things as caregivers: gastric tube feedings, doctors' visits, food swallowed by mouth, tumor markers, etc. I used three steno notebooks: one to track feedings (time and amount), one to track general overall condition (appearance, attitude, vocalizations, etc.), and one for "problems" with the long-term care facility.

I used a three-ring binder broken down with a tab for each doctor, so there was a section for the oncologist, neurologist, gastroenterologist, cardiologist, physical therapist, and speech therapist. That way, I always knew what one was doing, in case another one asked—I never relied upon doctor-to-doctor communication—and could always tell one doc what another one said. I would also use the binder to write questions down in advance of a doctor's visit, because you can't remember when you are there with the doctor.

My father did handle the billing and paperwork. I used to say that finally his MBA came in handy!! He would have one file dedicated to the EOBs and another one for the bills. He would match up the EOB to the bill to ensure that it was accurate. After he paid the bill, he would print out a copy of the paid check and attach all three together and file by doctor and date. He learned that it took about three medical bills before the amount due was correct. It did take time, but it is worth it; there was and still continues to be a lot of "double billing."

—Rich Ehrmann

{ Advance Directives }

by Kairol Rosenthal

Living wills are the coolest thing that nobody is doing. Do you want a living will? Chances are yes. Do you have a living will? Chances are no. I know this because I spent three years traipsing around the U.S. chatting with a plethora of young adult survivors for a book I wrote called *Everything Changes*. I talked to Muslims, Catholics, Jews, atheists, Baptists—all young, all with cancer; and most all of them would like a living will.

A living will is a legal document that informs your family and doctors about your wishes for medical treatment should you no longer be able to speak on your own behalf. (Remember Terri Schiavo, the Florida woman who, as she remained in a vegetative state, became a symbol for whether or not to take someone off life support?) It is a completely separate and different document from your last will and testament, in which you decide who gets your iPod and favorite sweatshirt when you kick the bucket.

A partner to the living will is a document called a medical power of attorney, aka health-care power of attorney. This document allows you to appoint a friend or family member to make decisions on your behalf. Together the living will and medical power of attorney make up what are known as advance directives.

Confused? Don't be. Here is the cheat sheet version: Advance directives are the umbrella. Underneath this umbrella are two documents

> **Get free downloadable advance directive forms, easy enough for a first grader, from www.Caringinfo.org.**

that make a fantastic duo: the living will and medical power of attorney.

Living will—Think "will," a document that states your wishes, in this case about your medical treatment.

Medical power of attorney—Think "attorney": An attorney is a human being (though some would argue that) who represents another, so the medical power of attorney is the document that states what human being in your life you want to make medical decisions on your behalf.

In a dark, dark room, in a dark, dark closet, in a dark, dark box, in a dark, dark envelope, I have legal advance directives. I hammered out the appropriate forms on the way to the hospital four hours before going under the knife. You can do it, too, and here is all you have to know: Advance directives scribbled on the back of a Starbucks receipt don't hold water. You must complete very simple legal papers, which vary from state to state and require a few signatures.

Note: If you are an interstate hospital-hopper, following a boyfriend across state lines or transferring to your third college across the country, you'll need to complete advance directives for each state in which you receive care on your cancer tour. Also, if you designated your BFF, boyfriend, girlfriend, fiancée, or spouse as your medical power of attorney and he or she has now for whatever reason moved to your shit list, you will want to make sure you name someone else.

There are a million reasons to procrastinate on writing advance directives. None of them are good. A common kvetch is, "What are the chances I'll really need them anyway?" I am sure if Terri Schiavo could, she'd change all the bumper stickers from "Shit Happens" to "Vegetative States Happen." Besides, if you are reading this book, chances are your medical track record kinda sucks to begin with, so why take your chances at the roulette wheel now?

Do it for yourself, do it for Terri, do it for your friends and family who will, let's hope, never have to scratch their heads wondering if they should pull a Kevorkian on you. After you've signed your advance directives, feel proud, dust off your khaki uniform, and sew on your newest cancer merit badge. You've earned it.

A Brief Tidbit about Your Workplace

We covered advance directives above, which make your wishes known to doctors and loved ones. In a way, you'll need to do the same thing with your employer. As you go about that likely delicate process, it's helpful to know what your employer is or isn't obligated to do after you're diagnosed. The first thing for you to know is that cancer *can* be a disability under the Americans with Disabilities Act (ADA).

According to the excellent Cancer and Careers Web site (www.cancerandcareers.org), the definition of a disability is "a physical or mental impairment that substantially impacts a major life activity." These days, major life activities include not only walking, talking, and breathing, but also sleeping, thinking, and communicating. Yes, the wheels of progress are screaming.

What does this mean regarding your job? Much of it boils down to the predictably lackluster term "reasonable accommodations." Your employer has to make reasonable accommodations for your cancer diagnosis. *Has to*—so long as it's not an undue hardship. Reasonable accommodations in your case can include reassignment to a vacant position, flexible hours, and/or an extended period of leave.

You have to request whatever reasonable accommodation you want, however; your employer isn't required to keep asking you if there's anything more you need. And finally, such requests are to be kept confidential, and your employer can request medical documentation that shows you need the accommodation and that you can perform the job safely if given the accommodation.

Insurance (and More!)

I have two private insurance companies and for four months—since my diagnosis—I have not been able to get either to pay for anything. All I have is a stack of unpaid bills and a laundry list of phone calls to make to figure out why they won't help.

—TYLER

It's probably too late to insist that you get health insurance and never let it lapse, but just in case: *Always have health insurance and never let*

> There are tests that perform gene analysis in an attempt to determine people's susceptibility to cancer (mostly BRCA tests, which analyze the likelihood of one's getting breast or ovarian cancer). This relates to insurance in the following way: Federal law now makes it impossible for health insurers to deny coverage or raise premiums based on BRCA status, but life insurers can.

it lapse. Not life insurance, but health insurance. (Life insurance pays a dollar amount to a designated beneficiary upon a policyholder's death; health insurance pays things like hospital fees and drug costs.)

Nearly seventy thousand young adults in the United States are diagnosed with cancer each year, and this number sadly includes too many without health insurance. The young adult population is the largest and fastest-growing group of uninsured and underinsured people in the U.S. Currently about thirteen million young adults are left wanting in the insurance arena. Forty percent of college graduates go without insurance for some time. The health-care changes motivated by the bill passed in March 2010, which allows young adults to remain on their parents' insurance until they are twenty-six, should help reduce these numbers.

If you're already in the shit without insurance, keep in mind the old adage: "If you can't be a good example, be a horrible warning." Tell all your friends to get insurance. Premiums on an individual health insurance plan (meaning a plan that you get on your own, not through a job) for healthy, noncancerous young adults can run from $50 to $200 a month. Forget how many drinks that would buy at your favorite club—it's worth it for even a bare-bones major medical plan in the event of a one-in-a-million catastrophe. Not that you'd know anything about rare medical catastrophes.

Insurance can help prevent a delayed diagnosis and can also prevent a post-diagnosis financial crisis with long-term repercussions. Try finding an individual insurance policy with a $100 premium after you've been diagnosed: Rates skyrocket to prohibitive levels.

Even if you have insurance, you still need to be organized, knowledgeable, and a giant, inexorable pain in the ass. To insurance companies in general, you're best when you're not pestering them about this and that reimbursement or demanding to know why such and such wasn't paid. If you don't have your facts at hand, you might get screwed.

So, if you have insurance, prepare yourself for some fun back-and-forth with your insurer regarding coverage. If you don't, prepare to wade through quicksand-y bureaucracy in search of some form of financial assistance.

Bottom line in either case: Gear up. Prepare to be your own best advocate. Get unlimited minutes on your phone (or get a landline), and get used to writing everything down. And make this your mantra: persistence, persistence, persistence.

Insurance Alphabet Soup

Following are descriptions of a few terms and services you've doubtless heard of, but whose particular purposes you might not be able to define.

> If you've been blindsided financially by your diagnosis, don't forget that each state has a program that provides free or low-cost insurance for kids (under eighteen) with hard-hit families. It covers things such as medical, dental, and hospital costs, as well as prescription medications. The criteria for qualification can change, so check out your state's program at www.insurekidsnow.gov.

As you navigate the financial side of Planet Cancer—marked by various unforeseen mountains and sinkholes—it's helpful to know what things like COBRA, HIPAA, Medicaid, and the Family Medical Leave Act are. They're defined below. It's a little dense, and the length and frequency of sidebars make this section appear as if David Foster Wallace had a hand in its creation, but don't skip it; this stuff is important!

A quick shout-out: Much of the information about insurance comes to us from the incredibly awesome crew at the **Patient Advocate Foundation (www.patientadvocate.org),** which helps safeguard people diagnosed with life-threatening or debilitating diseases by providing information and assistance for access to care, continued employment, and preservation of their financial stability. That's right: They do good.

What Is Medicaid?

Medicaid (not to be confused with Medicare) is a federally funded, state-regulated program that provides health-care coverage for certain categories of people with low incomes: children, parents of eligible kids, pregnant women, and the disabled. Which might be you (or your children). You can learn about Medicaid at your local health department or social service agency or, unsurprisingly, at your state's Medicaid office. Also try the social worker at your hospital. If you want to research it online, check out Medicaid eligibility criteria at www.cms.hhs.gov.

When you apply for Medicaid, *go in person* and take proof of income, proof of your diagnosis, and your doctors' contact information. (For a foolproof list of everything to take with you when you're going to stand in line for any treatment-related service, see later in the chapter.) There are countless programs in each state, and nobody knows them all, so don't let an eligibility worker tell you over the phone that you're ineligible or deter you from apply-

> Don't gloss over spend downs/cost shares! The Medically Needy Program is a Medicaid program that can help with your expenses, even if your income or assets exceed the limits for regular Medicaid. Each month, certain medical expenses called "allowable medical expenses" that you owe or have paid during the month count toward your spend down, which is calculated using your payments over a base period of a number of months. When the amount of allowable medical expenses is equal to your spend down, you become eligible for Medicaid for the rest of the month. Think of spend down like an insurance deductible, but with a name that sounds as if you're running a tab at a local canteen.

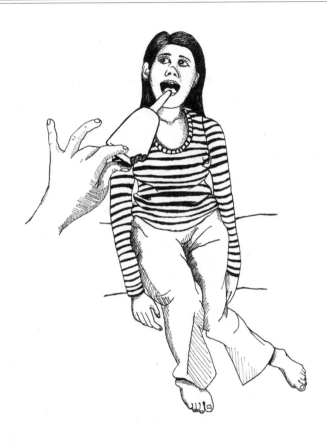

Top 10 Signs You've Joined a Cheap HMO

10. Annual breast exams are conducted at Hooters.

9. Directions to your doctor's office include, "Take a left when you enter the trailer park."

8. Tongue depressors taste faintly of Fudgesicles.

7. The colon specialist is only available on his days off from Roto-Rooter.

6. Only item listed under preventive care coverage is "An apple a day."

5. The used needle receptacles have recycling symbols on them.

4. "Patient responsible for 200 percent of out-of-network charges" is not a typo.

3. Your Prozac comes in different colors with little "m's" on them.

2. The radiation techs are wearing old Storm-trooper costumes.

1. The only expense covered 100 percent is embalming.

ing. *Note:* If you're approved for Supplemental Security Income (SSI), you're eligible for Medicaid. (SSI helps aged, blind, and disabled people—cancer can indeed be a disability—with little or no income by giving them cash for basic needs such as food, clothing, and shelter.)

To kick-start your practice of writing everything down, make sure that you get the name of the Medicaid worker who will handle your case. (And his or her birthday and favorite candy. We're just sayin'.)

If you're under nineteen years old—wait, why are you reading this? Just kidding—you could qualify for the State Children's Health Insurance Program (SCHIP). SCHIP requires states to provide health insurance to children from working families with incomes too high to qualify for Medicaid but too low to afford private health insurance. It provides coverage for medical services, prescription drugs, vision, hearing, and mental health services, and SCHIP is available everywhere. Your state Medicaid agency can provide more information about SCHIP, or you can read about it online at www.insurekidsnow.gov. You can also call (877) 543-7669.

What Is Medicare?

Though Medicare is typically associated with its role in helping pay health-care costs for people age sixty-five and older, it also helps people under age sixty-five with long-term disabilities—you know, like cancer.

Medicare can also be an option for young adults who have received Social Security Disability Income (SSDI) for a period of twenty-four consecutive months and for those with end-stage renal disease (permanent kidney fail-

ure treated with dialysis or a transplant). Or Lou Gehrig's disease, in case you are really, really, *really* unlucky.

To learn more, visit www.medicare.gov or call (800) MEDICARE (800-633-4227).

What Is COBRA?

The unfortunate acronym COBRA (how far away from warm and fuzzy could they get, really?) stands for the Consolidated Omnibus Budget Reconciliation Act, which applies to health insurance provided by an employer with more than twenty employees. COBRA allows your health insurance to continue after you:

- Leave a job

- Have your hours reduced

- Reach the age limit on your parents' insurance

Note: Some states offer mini-COBRA options to those who don't meet the guidelines of COBRA. The amount of coverage varies, depending on your state, and you must contact the insurer directly to enroll.

As long as your employer hasn't ended its insurance plan, you can continue to receive benefits for up to eighteen months after the insurance would have otherwise ended. (See the next entry, "Extending COBRA," and "If You Have to Quit Working" later in the chapter.) COBRA isn't insurance itself; it allows you to keep paying for the insurance you already have.

The downside: You have to pay the full premium on the plan, plus a 2 percent administrative fee, which can be pretty expensive. The upside: That's a lot cheaper than a new policy would be for the new, "cancer-improved" you. Plus, benefits under the plan shouldn't change. If you choose to continue coverage under COBRA, you start paying the premiums immediately after your coverage ends and continue as long as you want to receive benefits, up to eighteen months. In other words, once you stop COBRA, you can't start it back up. (You can also extend up to thirty-six months in the case of divorce. Call it the "Good News/Bad News" clause.)

Once COBRA benefits have been exhausted, hello world! Your best option is to get a job with an employer that offers group health coverage. As long as there's not a sixty-three-day (or longer) lapse in insurance coverage, you can enroll into a new employer policy without being subject to any preexisting clauses, regardless of previous health conditions (see next section, "What Is HIPAA?").

The health-care bill passed in March 2010 prohibits insurers from considering preexisting conditions in people under nineteen years old. (This includes insurers imposing waiting periods regarding preexisting conditions, such as when you switch jobs. Before the change, insurance companies could slap a waiting period of up to a year on anyone switching insurance coverage.) For those older than nineteen, the same rules regarding preexisting conditions go into effect in 2014. So if you're older than ninteen and sixty-three days or more elapse without coverage, you're still eligible for employer-sponsored coverage, but a twelve-month preexisting condition clause may be applied until changes go into effect in 2014. This means you can access the health-care benefits offered through the plan except those treatments and/or therapies related to a preexisting condition (like your cancer, for instance) for twelve months. After those twelve months the plan has to cover your preexisting condition (see "What Is HIPAA?"). If you enter the private individual insurance market after COBRA, the sixty-three-day lapse becomes more important, because until 2014, there aren't any protections for preexisting conditions in the individual insurance market—until then, insurers can continue to deny coverage, or at least leave your preexisting condition(s) out of individual policies.

So we'll say it again here: *Don't let your coverage lapse!*

Check out COBRA online: www.dol.gov/dol/topic/health-plans/cobra.htm and www.cobra health.com, where the very first thing you'll see as of this writing is this: "We know the COBRA regulations can be confusing and contradicting." Enjoy!

Extending COBRA

In certain circumstances your COBRA can be extended for eleven months. Without explaining these circumstances—each case is unique, and do you really want us to use phrases like "second qualifying event"?—here's what we

---

Some states offer HIPAA individual plans. To learn about your state's offerings, contact your Department of Insurance or visit www.insure.com/articles/healthinsurance/HIPAA.html.

need to stress: The cost during the extension period can jump from 102 percent of the cost of coverage, which it is during the initial period, to 150 percent. Sadly, this might be a better option than the alternative. Like having nothing.

What Is HIPAA?

HIPAA stands for the Health Insurance Portability and Accountability Act (1996), which protects rights related to health insurance. The "portability" part of the law prohibits a group plan from excluding people or raising premiums based on individuals' health history or disability. So HIPAA applies only to insurance you get through a job, not individual plans.

If you're starting a new job and have been without insurance for more than sixty-three days—ominously known as a "significant break"—and you are older than nineteen, a group plan can exclude coverage for anything cancer-related (or, for that matter, for any other preexisting condition you might have) until 2014. HIPAA says that a plan can only do that for up to twelve months, after which it has to cover anything related to your preexisting conditions. HIPAA also keeps your medical information confidential, so your boss can't get it from your doctor without your permission.

To learn more about your protections under HIPAA, visit www.dol.gov/topic/health-plans/portability.htm.

If You Don't Have Insurance

Don't panic if this eighteen-wheeler hits you and you're not covered. (See "What It's Really Like to . . . Go through Treatment without Insurance" later in the chapter.)

Organizations that offer charity care and/or financial assistance are out there; you just have to find them. Start by asking your doctor and your local hospital whether they offer assistance; if not, the hospital contact (social worker, patient advocate, or financial counselor) can tell you which ones do and may also give you other local resources for direct financial assistance.

Ask your hospital contact for an application for **charity care/financial assistance.** Typically, assistance organizations base eligibility on income, assets, and household size; requirements for qualifying vary. Some offer 100 percent charity care. Others use a sliding-scale fee based on your income.

With charity care, hospital charges will be covered, but providers will bill separately— you'll need to make separate arrangements with them. Occasionally, if the hospital is doing a charity write-off for your care, the providers will follow suit. If charity care isn't available, discuss payment arrangements with the provider.

Another option is to access your state's **Hill-Burton facilities,** if available. These facilities provide limited care to uninsured patients whose income meets certain requirements, usually based on U.S. Department of Health and

---

Risk pools offer insurance to those turned down by individual plans or who have been offered plans with elimination riders or very high premiums. To find out more, check out www.healthinsurance.org/risk_pools.

Human Services Poverty Guidelines. To locate a Hill-Burton facility in your area, call (800) 638-0742 or check out www.hrsa.gov/hillburton/hillburtonfacilities.htm.

Additionally, some states offer county medical assistance for those who don't qualify for Medicaid but are still underserved. If you don't qualify for Medicaid, find out from your local social services representative whether your county offers such assistance.

Beginning January 1, 2014, health insurance exchanges will be established in each state. The exchanges will first open to the individual and small group markets and will allow the purchase of health insurance coverage with guaranteed issue, no preexisting conditions, elimination of annual/lifetime limits on coverage, and caps on out-of-pocket expenses. Until then, part of the health bill passed in early 2010 is a high-risk insurance pool, which will offer subsidized premiums to people who have been uninsured for at least six months and have yet-to-be-defined medical problems.

Be Prepared When You're Applying for Assistance
(Or, Don't Waste Your Time in Line)

If you're going after assistance, here's what sucks: waiting in line for hours, getting to the front of the line, and being sent away because you don't have everything you need for your application. The list below, compiled by the Patient Advocate Foundation, will make you the envy of everyone in line. Put these documents in a folder and keep them with you whenever you enter administrative mode.

Some of the items are specific to certain requests, such as applying for disability. The financial items, however, along with your birth certificate, driver's license, and Social Security card are required to apply for most programs (and often are required for the entire family if applying for federal or state programs).

The Solid-Gold, Ready-for-Anything, I Will Not Be Sent Away from This Line Empty-handed List!

- Income tax returns for the past two years. If you didn't file income tax returns, then they typically need your two most recent W-2 forms or last six pay stubs from your employer.

- Number in the household (regarding things like food stamps, the concern here is how many mouths there are to feed in the house; for a public assistance budget that might help with rent, they're interested in who's contributing to household income).

- If you are receiving (or paying) income from another source, such as Social Security, retirement, alimony, child support, VA, welfare, etc., provide documentation for verification.

- Two or three recent bank statements.

- Notification of Benefit Decision from the Department of Health and Human Services

> Contrary to popular belief, unpaid hospital medical bills do not affect your credit standing. The bill collectors may be annoying, and large bills could go into litigation, but your credit score is safe. This is because reporting to credit agencies is a voluntary process, and hospitals generally don't do it. That said, many smaller clinics and labs do report delinquent payments to collection agencies; such agencies don't differentiate between unpaid medical bills and, say, cell phone bills, so if your unpaid medical bills find their way to them, your credit score could actually be affected.

> { If you create a system in which one person's life depends upon their ex-coworker faxing a letter, the system deserves to be rattled. }

(if applicable), such as a Medicaid denial or award.

- Proof of expenses (copies).

- Rent/mortgage bills or letter from landlord, and all utility bills (cable, phone, electric, gas, etc.), including those from a second property.

- Other medical bills.

- Proof of payment for vehicle or vehicles (also the ages, makes, and models—include items such as boats, motorcycles, motor homes, land, vacation property, etc.).

- Any bill you are paying right now (child care, student loans, etc.).

- Copy of your birth certificate (originals are needed on occasion to verify authenticity);

you'll need to provide birth certificates for all members of the family if applying for federal or state assistance.

- Social Security card (for all members of the family if applying for federal or state assistance).

- Driver's license.

- Name, address, and phone number for the treating physician(s) and hospitals, labs, clinics, etc.

- If insured, name of insurer, identification number and phone number, type of coverage (plan language or link, username, and password to plan online).

- Medical records (if available, having these saves time); typically needed for disability applications.

- Letter of support from your physician; typically needed for disability applications.

- List of medications that you're taking.

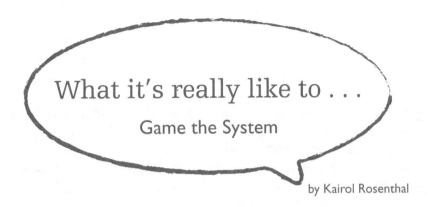

What it's really like to . . .

Game the System

by Kairol Rosenthal

If I told you that I'm not proud of the lies I have told, well, I'd be lying. It wasn't courage or bravery that landed me a spot on the surgery table; it was fudged health insurance. As equally frightening as surgery was the possibility that, while I was under the knife, the insurance company would realize my coverage was a sham.

What was even more surprising than the words "you have cancer" was the medical receptionist's response when I tried to schedule a second opinion: "You have no insurance." I had left my job three weeks before, and the human resources director, who shared my office, forgot to submit my COBRA papers.

I have heard stories of women who, when their children are trapped under a car, become possessed with Herculean strength. They will hoist a three-thousand-pound vehicle to save their kid's life. I was suddenly the mother and the kid at once. I needed the best medical care possible and would do anything to get it. My cancer fight was not fueled by the kind of strength you see written about on a pink Hallmark cancer card. My strength was super-human, fueled by adrenaline. My humility, dignity, and honesty evaporated quickly. Staging a one-woman sit-in, I returned to the small art museum where I had been employed and refused to leave the director's office until she remedied the situation.

Her apologies felt like empty insults. "I'm sorry" would not pay for anesthesia, a hospital bed, or treatment. On my third trip to her office, she offered to lie to the insurance company, telling them I had returned to work so my coverage could be reinstated. This was far from a perfect solution. It was illegal. I explained to her that the insurance company could perform an audit, discover I was no longer on the payroll, and my insurance could be canceled immediately. "What are the chances that will happen?" she asked. "What are the chances I'd be sitting in your office with cancer?" I replied. To buy myself time, I accepted her offer and left.

My employer's scam covered me through the next few weeks of second and third opinions. My final appointment was with the top thyroid cancer surgeon in the United States, whose practice happened to be in my city. His schedule was booked for a month. I waited, filling my days with my new full-time job of sitting on the phone from 8:30 to 4:30 with the national COBRA headquarters in Florida.

There are some things that a college education will never teach you: shrewdness, persistence, and manipulation. When speaking with Violet, an operator at COBRA, I used my mother's advice that honey goes further than vinegar. In chatty conversation, Violet told me she was the mother of three. I told her how much I missed my mom, who lived across the country, and how I wished she could hold my hand through every day of cancer. I almost got Violet to cry, but more importantly I got her to give me her direct phone number.

I worked Violet for days on end, asking casual questions, milking from her the names and department locations of higher-ups in the COBRA administration and learning the code names and protocols for emergency administrative procedures.

I was two-timing Violet. On calls with dozens of other operators and supervisors, I was harsh and demanding. I fabricated a missing paper trail initiated by higher-ups whom I had never actually spoken with, and I blamed others, whom I had also never contacted, for the disappearance of these nonexistent papers.

As though my life had become a James Bond movie, the COBRA procedure I needed was called Code Red. Through my web of lies, I procured a Code Red approval and was on COBRA just in time for surgery. After surgery and before treatment, I hunted for resources and advice to shore up my COBRA coverage. A student at a law school clinic helped me gain a legal, eighteen-month extension of my COBRA.

Three years later, while researching a book I wrote on young adult cancer, I discovered that many organizations provide insurance counseling to cancer patients. Yet, I learned, even the best counselors are able to procure insurance for patients in only a small minority of cases. Our system is flawed beyond repair, and this is why I still feel no guilt about my cunning lies. If you create a system in which one person's life depends upon their ex-coworker faxing a letter, the system deserves to be rattled.

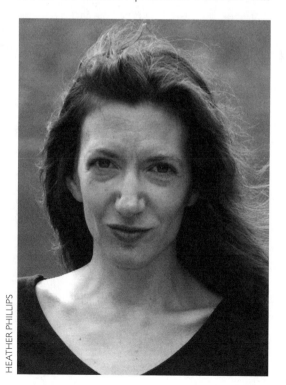

HEATHER PHILLIPS

Guides to the Planet

Kairol Rosenthal is the author of *Everything Changes: The Insider's Guide to Cancer in Your 20s and 30s* (Wiley, 2009). She was diagnosed with thyroid cancer at twenty-seven. After surgery and radioactive iodine treatment, Kairol hit the road with tape recorder in hand. From the Big Apple to the Bible Belt, she became a one-woman cancer confessional, recording the intimate stories of twenty- and thirtysomething survivors. *Everything Changes* details her travels and includes unprecedented young adult cancer resources.

Kairol is cohost of *The Stupid Cancer Show.* She is a prolific blogger: Visit www.every thingchangesbook.com.

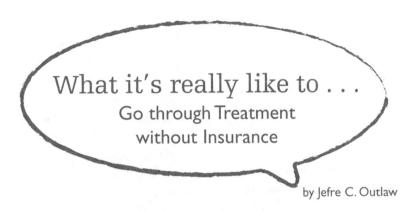

What it's really like to . . .
Go through Treatment
without Insurance

by Jefre C. Outlaw

In 2004 I wasn't feeling well. I did not go to a doctor because I had no health insurance. Money was tight, my savings minuscule. I became very angry, and I blamed others for my misfortune. On December 1, 2004, a pain in my side started that would not go away. I did not sleep for four days. For fear of passing out behind the wheel of my truck, I made it a priority to see my regular doctor. She became very concerned and set me up for a CT scan. I could not pay for it that day, so I paid $100 and set up a payment plan with the radiology clinic. The results showed a softball-size mass in my abdomen that explained the pain. The specialists said, "It could be anything." They knew full well it had to be cancer.

I spent the next month and all my savings getting more tests. On January 5, 2005, I heard the diagnosis: Stage III advanced aggressive non-Hodgkin's lymphoma, large B-cell CD 20 positive. Strange how we cancer survivors remember these dates and all the diagnostic details. Our lives change forever when we hear those words.

Hearing the oncologist say that if you don't respond to aggressive treatment you'll be dead by the end of the year—that will hit you hard. Treatment would cost $220,000. These words turned my life upside down. Like many young people, I lived hand to mouth. Moreover, I had just spent all my savings to get diagnosed. Uncertainty compounded. Where was this headed?

Left with few choices and no family support, I turned my house over to the lender. I turned my car in to the lender. I turned myself into a live-in with a gracious friend from church. My household contents were put in a storage unit; thieves cut the lock and took it all. Next, my contract job let me go due to my cancer diagnosis, and Social Security Disability Insurance turned my application down twice! Adding to the pain, my girlfriend walked out on me, as she could not deal with the emotional side of all of this. I do not blame her. We had not been dating long, and cancer was really heavy stuff.

To recap: I lost my health, I lost my home, I lost my car, my household contents, my job, and my girlfriend. It sounds like a country-western song! Perhaps I should write one.

In a span of four months, I had been left with a mattress, some clothes, my laptop, and my two dogs. No money, no way to work, and no way to get treatment. Wow! What a housecleaning God had in store for me! So, here I am sleeping on a mattress thrown down on my friend's dining room floor. My friend was in Brazil for three months, so I was on my own. The pain was so bad I did not sleep for days. I remember one morning not being able to get the toaster to work. The plugs in the kitchen were

59

> **Neuropathy:** when a peripheral nerve works poorly, is damaged, etc. Your limbs might feel weak or numb if you suffer from neuropathy.

not working, and I could not find a bad breaker. So I set up the toaster in the bathroom and from that point forward the bathroom always smelled like toast. I must have been delusional from the pain.

Social workers at the clinic where I was diagnosed put me in contact with welfare resources including the Medical Assistance Program (MAP) coordinators. Since I had less than $500 in assets, I qualified for welfare and food stamps. This included medical care through the county Medical Assistance Program: basically, care for the homeless. Apparently most large counties have some kind of property tax-funded program like this that funds the county hospital for indigent care. The big pharmaceutical companies also donate drugs for the treatment of people in MAP. Getting approved required several interviews and lots of paperwork. But, to their credit, they did not hold up my treatment.

I received six very expensive cycles of R-CHOP at the county hospital from very loving and caring people at no cost to me. I felt like the doctors, nurses, and other staff were as good if not better than any care I could have received elsewhere. They dealt with a lot of people who were in very poor health to begin with, so I was a cream puff for them, as I was in generally very good health except for the cancer. The standard of care was no different for me than for anyone with insurance.

The chemo treatments were harsh, as they all are. I had a loss of energy and some infections, and I lost my hair. But thanks to using combined therapy—western medicine and eastern/holistic medicine—I avoided most side effects. Acupunc-

ture each day after the chemo kept me from being nauseated. Massage therapy helped keep the neuropathy to almost nonexistent levels. Energy work helped to keep me positive and upbeat about this life experience and helped me clear a lot of negative stuff from my mind. Detox foot baths at my chiropractor's office helped me remove the chemo toxins from my body. My naturopath gave me supplements to help replenish my body with the vitamins and minerals that the chemo was stripping away. The life coach helped me focus on the positive and got me to start envisioning myself being well and living the life of my dreams. How did I pay for all this stuff? Well, my friends held twelve fundraisers, raising over $20,000 that was used for incidental expenses. My church set up a tax-free donation fund and accepted donations for my care.

I had a massage therapist, energy worker, chiropractor, acupuncturist, life coach, and naturopath all donate their services to treat me with alternative care—people who taught me how to forgive and heal my spirit. Simultaneously, I received conventional western medicine at the local hospital. It was an amazing experience. I went into remission and stopped my chemo treatments a month early. I had my health back—my most precious

> Visit www.needymeds.org to be linked to any available disease-specific co-pay programs and any free or reduced-cost patient assistance programs for pharmaceutical prescription needs. Also, many large pharmacy chains like Wal-Mart, Target, and Walgreens have started offering generic medications at very low prices.

resource—and no medical debt to speak of. The key was working closely with the welfare and MAP providers to make sure that all the neces-sary paperwork was filled out so that I qualified for indigent care. I had no choice but to make myself indigent to get treatment.

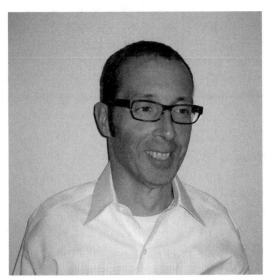

Guides to the Planet

Jefre C. Outlaw was diagnosed with non-Hodgkin's lymphoma (NHL) at age forty-two. Although the diagnosis and intensive chemo-therapy subsequently turned his life into a country song, he reached remission nonetheless. Four years later, the NHL relapsed, and Jefre underwent a stem cell transplant to cure his cancer. He lives in Austin, Texas, and lives his life in the spirit of paying it forward.

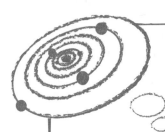

Dispatches from the Planet

I had a private nurse come to my home after my mastectomy/reconstruction, and my insurance covered it! I would have *never* thought to call if I hadn't heard about that from a friend of mine. I have learned that many insurance policies will cover "thera-peutic massage" through a physical thera-pist. There are many holistic/complementary types of therapies out there to aid in your healing and wellness, but you need to check around and *ask, ask,* and *ask* some more. There are even cancer camps out there!

—Amy L. Paradise

Other Insurance Issues

If you are lucky enough to have insurance, congratulations! The odds that you actually would have to use your policy were slim, but wow is it ever worth it now. Cancer without insurance is its own special circus of trials, but having insurance is not all sunshine and ambrosia. Following are a couple of prickly situations that you might encounter even with an insurance policy:

If Your Policy Is Maxed Out

Apply for Medicaid. When you apply, Medicaid might ask you to provide proof that your LTM (lifetime maximum) has been exhausted. Typically this is done via a letter from your insurance company.

Other options: Change employment or enroll into a risk pool plan, if available, in your state of residence. With a new health plan, your lifetime maximum starts over at zero.

Taking these options entails some downside, such as likely higher premiums and the potential for a lapse of coverage, which would bring your cancer into play with your new policy.

If Your Policy Is Inadequate

In the case of your policy not covering all your costs, Medicaid can become a secondary insurance. The local Medicaid office will need verification of your primary insurance coverage. Also, if your pharmacy coverage is minimal, there are co-payment assistance programs available. (*Note:* You're not eligible to apply for these assistance programs if you don't have some sort of pharmacy coverage to begin with.)

Family Medical Leave Act (FMLA)

If you're covered through work, your company is most likely paying part of your premium—customarily more than half. So coverage isn't such a big issue for you, but it's possible that working will be. You might want to take some time off, work reduced hours, or otherwise alter your traditional, noncancer schedule. With that in mind, here's the Family Medical Leave Act.

The act allows employees to take up to twelve weeks of unpaid leave during a twelve-month period. Leave can be taken for your own health or to care for a family member, and can be continuous or intermittent—you know, like taking a day each week to go to doctor's appointments.

When your leave is completed, your employer must reinstate you to your original job or an equivalent one, with the same benefits and seniority. During the leave, you must be allowed to keep your health insurance on the same terms as when you were working, so you may have to make payments to your employer for the premiums that would normally be taken from your paycheck. Your employer may require you to exhaust your paid time off (including vacation and sick time) before taking FMLA leave.

FMLA-related correspondence and documentation should go through the human resources or benefits departments, or through your manager if your company doesn't have these positions. Stay in touch during your leave, and notify an appropriate contact person if any changes arise that may affect your leave.

FMLA applies to:

- Public agencies (including state, local, and federal employers) and local education agencies (schools)

- Private-sector employers who employ fifty or more employees in

twenty or more workweeks in the current or preceding calendar year

Many states have laws that improve upon FMLA requirements, and many companies have policies that provide more benefits than mandated by law. Be sure to check with your HR department or employee handbook to learn your company's policies. Regardless, be sure to talk with your doctors about the length and intensity of your treatment, to give written and verbal notice of your request for leave and its anticipated duration, and to fill out any required forms—something you're sure to be skilled at doing by the end of this process.

If You Have to Quit Working

If you lost your job or reduced your hours as a result of illness and are therefore no longer eligible for employee health insurance coverage, you may be eligible for eighteen months of COBRA coverage—with an extension option of eleven months if you're deemed disabled under COBRA guidelines.

Important and often misunderstood are the provisions around the eleven-month extension. Breathe deeply and read on. This extension is available if two criteria are met:

1. The qualified beneficiary is determined by the Social Security Administration to be disabled at some point before the sixtieth day of COBRA coverage.

2. The qualified beneficiary (or another person on his or her behalf) notifies the health plan administrator of the SSA determination within sixty days of receiving the award but prior to the end of COBRA coverage (eighteen months).

> Young adults are the demographic group most likely to be under- or uninsured. Many young adults are too old for their parents' insurance or government programs for kids, yet they are more likely not to be in established careers with full health benefits.

You can punish yourself more by reading the law in its entirety at www.cms.gov.

Some states have health insurance premium payment benefits under their Medicaid program. If you're eligible for coverage under a COBRA plan, your state may provide benefits in the form of premium payments and allow you to maintain current coverage rather than be covered by Medicaid. To find out if your state offers this benefit, contact your local Medicaid office.

If Your Premiums Are Raised

If you're part of a **group policy** and you think that your rates have increased while those of others in the group haven't, that's illegal. Monkey business along these lines merits a call to your state's Department of Insurance.

If you have an **individual insurance policy** and your premiums are raised, here's some news: Your policy isn't regulated. Boo. Group policies can raise premiums *only* if they raise them for the entire group. Individual policies can be raised at renewal time based on claims activity over the past year. Beginning in 2014, however, new rules regarding premiums will take effect. Premiums will no longer be allowed to be raised based on health status. Premiums will be varied based on age, tobacco use, geographic area, and family size.

{ The first thing to keep
in mind: You don't have
to be a mere passenger
on the treatment train. }

Chapter Three

Treatment

Man, I hated treatment. The upside: It made me love the shit out of everything else. I'm good at living now. I can't say that about myself pretreatment.

—HL1994

I have changed more in the last three years than I ever thought I'd change in my lifetime. Looking at me, you wouldn't know that. But deep inside, there has been a revolution that is hard to explain.

—CARTWHEELSKY

It hurts like fucking hell most of the time. But I think that hurt is just our hearts growing bigger and stronger, much like a muscle grows when it is worked out.

—DENNY

Hearing the words "you have cancer" is possibly the most out-of-control experience you will ever have. It's a UFO landing on your head, a dizzy-making sucker punch whose effects last for days—shocking, unbelievable, and, to understate it a bit, change-inducing. In the aftermath, after the sirens stop blaring, putting together a treatment plan is one of the first places you can regain control.

The first thing to keep in mind: You don't have to be a mere passenger on the treatment train. The medical team will make recommendations; then it's up to you and/or your team of trusted advisors to evaluate what you're being told, ask questions, and seek a second, third, even a fourth opinion. Your recommended treatment depends on lots of things, including the type of cancer, the stage, grade, tumor location, genetic profile, and even your age. Treatment may include chemotherapy, radiation, surgery, or any combination of the three.

However physically easy or hard the actual medical treatment may be—and it varies wildly from person to person—a cancer diagnosis is nearly guaranteed to upend every aspect of your life. So your treatment plan should go beyond the hospital and the doctors' offices to include everything else you do to support your own health and wellness.

Think long and hard about what you can bring to your treatment plan, to add to whatever is being transcribed into your rapidly expanding patient file. Maybe exercise makes you feel better, or you've been meaning to be more mindful about what you eat. Maybe you'd like to try massage, acupuncture, yoga, meditation, counseling, or simply knocking off work early some days. Anything that makes you stronger and better able to handle cancer treatment can be an important element of your treatment plan. (Read more about exercise, nutrition, and complementary and alternative medicine (CAM) in chapter 5.)

As you adjust to the Planet, your doctors are your coconspirators. Always let them know what

Stage describes how far cancer has spread. Overall stage groupings describe a cancer's stage with numerals I to IV: I indicates a localized tumor, and IV indicates metastatic cancer, or cancer that has spread.

Grade uses numerals I to IV to illustrate the aggressiveness of cancer cells (i.e., how fast they spread). Grade I (low-grade) is the least belligerent; IV (high-grade) is the most.

Don't be passive. Take control of your treatment and your body, and navigate the Planet with your own compass.

That said, your doctor does know you better than you might think. Too often, cancer patients enter treatment with little idea of how doctors attend to them. The popular misconception is that they zip through hospitals from patient to patient, dispensing standardized treatments, and speed off to the next place, dropping one patient file and grabbing another. Though some-

you're doing outside their four walls and keep them informed about what you're considering adding to your treatment plan, whether it's acupuncture, supplements, or an Alaskan cruise. We're not saying you have to get a permission slip—what are they going to do, ground you?—but full disclosure can't hurt, and it will help you avoid pitfalls and potential dangers.

Let's face it: This is your body, and your health is your responsibility. No one will ever know your body as well as you or have as much at stake in its healthy operation and maintenance.

> Don't be passive. Take control of your treatment and your body, and navigate the Planet with your own compass.

times this may be the case, we wanted to break down that wall, if slightly, by letting you read what a real oncologist does to prepare for meeting you for the first time.

What it's really like to . . .
Meet a Newly Diagnosed Cancer Patient

by Christian Cable, M.D. (aka Dr. Disco)

Meeting your oncologist for the first time is daunting for both of you. He or she is asking for your trust and giving you so much information so quickly that it feels as if you're drinking from a fire hose. Your collaboration begins at this visit, and you'll start with less information and experience than your doctor. A good physician recognizes that, nonetheless, you are the expert in you, and he or she cares about the support you'll need. Here's the thought process I follow when meeting a person with a new diagnosis of cancer:

1. Does my patient understand the diagnosis? If so, can I clarify anything? If not, how can I best educate him or her? Are family members and friends in attendance? I write things down and recommend Web sites that offer things in layman's or technical language. My go-to Web site is www.cancer.gov.

2. What is the stage of disease? Do we have further tests to do to determine the stage? Different stages of the same disease may be treated differently. Do we need PET scans, or would a CT scan or MRI be better?

3. Is there a well-established therapy to treat this cancer? I compare established treatments with clinical trials (see "Clinical Tri-

als" later in the chapter) and other attempts to improve on that therapy. For example, ABVD chemotherapy is standard treatment for most cases of Hodgkin's lymphoma. I will explore the availability of alternatives if consensus is not as strong to follow this standard treatment. (It's worth stressing here that most knowledge in breast cancer has been advanced via large clinical trials and that there is no "placebo" in a cancer-focused clinical trial that will give you less than the generally accepted standard of care.)

4. How healthy is my patient? The assumption that all young adults are healthy is as false as the assumption that all elderly are frail. I expect someone who has healthy eating and exercise habits to cope better with therapy. Some patients mark an interest in a healthy

---

ABVD chemotherapy combines Adriamycin, bleomycin, vinblastine, and DTIC in a four-horse chemo cocktail. Though we don't go into describing specific drugs in this book, you can find explanations of the various types of chemotherapeutic drugs in this chapter.

lifestyle from the time of cancer diagnosis, their good habits continuing after the cancer is long gone.

Integrating this information in an hour is a challenge. I make a treatment recommendation based on all of the above. I've done my homework on each patient before we meet so that I can understand the data we have and identify the information still needed.

I research new treatments or rare diseases by reviewing national treatment guidelines such as those issued by the NCCN (the National Comprehensive Cancer Network, an alliance of twenty-one leading cancer centers worldwide). I also attend national meetings in my specialty and attend the educational and scientific sessions appropriate to my patient population. Finally, I have a list of nationwide experts who have been very gracious to respond to my e-mail inquiries on difficult cases.

I feel an obligation to competence, but that isn't really the soul of cancer care to me. I like my patients and consider it a privilege to be on their team. So the first meeting is indeed an introduction that I cherish. It is the beginning of a relationship and a partnership, and it can make all the difference.

> I've done my homework on each patient before we meet so that I can understand the data we have and identify the information still needed.

Top 7 Signs Your Doctor May Be Coming on to You

This list, originally published on mcsweeneys.net, was shared with us by Wendy Molyneux, from her book *Everything Is Wrong with You: The Modern Woman's Guide to Finding Self Confidence through Self Loathing.*

7. He asks you to turn your head to the side and say, "I love you."

6. He Photoshops his picture onto an X-ray of your heart.

5. His lab coat says "Tight Butts Drive Me Nuts" on the back.

4. When you lie down on the examination table, he insists on spooning.

3. Before examining you, he washes his hands in Obsession by Calvin Klein.

2. He tells you that you have "sexy cancer."

1. While giving you a Pap smear, he "finds" an engagement ring.

Chemotherapy

Asked how long I had been going through chemo, I said a year. The lady said, "At your age, it must seem like yesterday."

No, it seemed like a friggin' year. I was there most of it.

—WILLIE B

Most people's hazy knowledge of chemotherapy comes from after-school specials showing amazingly continuous vomiting by a bald person. But "chemo," as it's not-so-affectionately called by insiders, is so much more.

Chemo is system-wide treatment that introduces toxic chemicals into your body, usually delivered by IV infusion. Chemo interrupts cell growth cycles: The hope is to catch cancer cells in mid-division and damage them beyond repair. Fast-growing cells are usually the most affected by chemo—in addition to cancer cells, the other most likely targets are in the hair, bone marrow, mouth, and intestinal tract. Thus, the telltale chemo signs of baldness, vomiting, and (less noticeable but more problematic) a drop in blood counts, as white blood cells, red blood cells, and platelets take hits for the team.

Fortunately, along with the development of more effective chemo drugs has come better ways of dealing with pesky side effects. New antinausea medications have significantly reduced offerings to the porcelain god, and there are shots that can turbocharge bone marrow production of red and white blood cells to keep patients out of the danger zone.

There are many different chemotherapy drugs, used in a variety of ways—some singly, some in various combinations—to treat different types of cancer. Dosages vary, methods of administration vary, schedules vary; it follows that even side effects vary: One person may hurl at the mere thought of chemo (anticipatory nausea), while another person on the same regimen munches jalapeño poppers during infusion with no ill effects. Some people lose their hair; others don't.

Bottom line: Although there are standard regimens for most types of cancer, every patient is an individual whose treatment will in some way be customized to his or her needs and circumstances. Whatever the customization, you can safely conclude that you're getting chemo for one of a few reasons:

1. **To cure you of cancer,** whether that means blasting your tumor (and the rest of your body: See "Side Effects" in chapter 4) with chemicals or a post-tumor-removal round to get rid of any lingering cancer cells.

2. **To control/reduce a tumor's growth** before another form of treatment, such as surgery or radiation.

3. Related to No. 2, to control a tumor's growth, but **simply to lessen the pain** that it might be causing.

It's important to understand which of those reasons brings you through the hospital doors into a place where you'll be surrounded by patients largely much older or younger than you. Communicate with your oncologist. Make sure you, your doctor, and your team of advisors are on the same page, both in what's coming and what to expect.

Once that's settled, you need to understand how your chemo will be delivered. Some chemo drugs come in pill form that you can swallow,

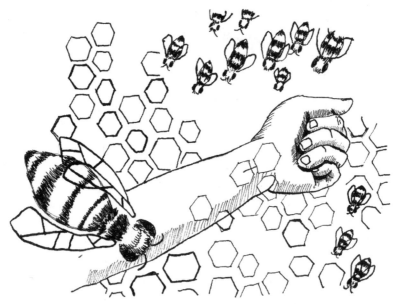

Top 10 Ways to Get a Taste of the Chemo Experience

From a Hodgkin's disease survivor, age twenty-two

10. Set down a delicious array of food before you, then eat only wood pulp for several days.

9. Throw up on your lawn.

8. Each week at a predetermined time, wake up, collect some bees, and let them sting you. (For that "I can't seem to get a vein" feeling, apply one of the little brutes to your arm with Scotch tape.)

7. Throw up on your neighbor's lawn.

6. Shave off your eyebrows, take out your eyelashes (except maybe three), then Nair the rest of your body. Don't worry—the burning is normal.

5. For that fun Ativan feeling, wander into a room and ponder all possible meanings of the word "amazing." Walk out of the room, repeat.

4. Hang upside down from a tree until your face is cherry red. Bingo: the dizzy, red-faced feeling of Adriamycin.

3. Lie around feeling as if you got hit by a truck.

2. Attempt to drink Ensure while you are nauseated. To become nauseated, drink an Ensure.

1. Congratulate yourself! You've finished one round of chemo. How many more you got?

some come via shots (both short- and long-needled: Needle size is determined by whether the chemo needs to go under the skin or into the muscle), but most chemo delivery still takes place as you see in the movies: intravenously, via catheters (see "Fun with Catheters" in chapter 2).

Types of Chemotherapy Drugs

by Cambrey Thomas

Now that you know how you're getting your chemotherapy, it only makes sense to examine what it is that's being pumped into you, or what you're swallowing or injecting.

Alkylating Agents

If cancer were a stalker, then alkylating agents would be the restraining order. Alkylating agents stop cancer cells from reproducing by causing a mutation that inhibits their DNA from splitting into a double helix. As the DNA is unable to split, the cell stops functioning.

Cornelius P. Rhoads discovered the properties of alkylating agents during World War II when a German air raid on an Italian harbor sank American ships and caused the ships' stores of nitrogen mustard gas to be released. Rhoads realized that the sailors exposed to the gas all had significantly low levels of white blood cells, which prompted him to use the agents to treat leukemia.

Alkylating agents, particularly carmustine, are still used in the treatment of leukemia, Hodgkin's disease, and other tumors. (Other examples are cyclophosphamide, ifosfamide, and cisplatin.) Most cancer treatments do not break the blood-brain barrier, but alkylating agents may be able to cross over. Helloooo, chemo brain (see chapter 4).

Antimetabolites

A case of mistaken identity is the catalyst for this mole of a cancer drug. Antimetabolites such as methotrexate, 5-fluorouracil, and gemcitabine work by fooling cells into using them as metabolites, which are the agents that help cells make nucleic acid. Once the antimetabolites are inside, the duped cancer cells die. Antimetabolites are taken orally. They can cause nausea, mouth sores, rashes, low blood counts, and abnormal liver function.

Anticancer Antibiotics

It doesn't always pay to be the fastest one at the race. Just like penicillin, anticancer antibiotics block the synthesis of DNA and RNA in rapidly dividing cells. The pro of this fungus-based drug, whose membership includes doxorubicin, dactinomycin, and bleomycin, is that it targets rapidly dividing cancer cells. The con is that it does not discriminate, so it can kill off healthy blood cells too. Anticancer antibiotics are given intravenously.

In most of your body, the smallest blood vessels, called capillaries, allow for easy transfer of many substances (glucose, for example) between the outside and inside of the vessels. In the blood-brain barrier, the cells that allow for this transfer are packed tightly together. They're more selective as to what can pass through, the goal being, of course, to protect the brain.

They motivate the classic chemo side effects: hair loss, nausea, and low platelets.

Plant Alkaloids

Periwinkle and Asian Happy Tree don't sound threatening in the fight against cancer, but extracts from these plants are, in fact, pugnacious cancer drugs with very different names: vincristine, docetaxel, etoposide, irinotecan.

Administered intravenously, plant alkaloids work by stopping cell functions as the cell enters the mitosis phase. Not only does the cell die, but it dies before it can reproduce. Although that sounds like a positive, plant alkaloids are unable to tell between cancerous and noncancerous cells. Opium was the first successful alkaloid isolated from a plant.

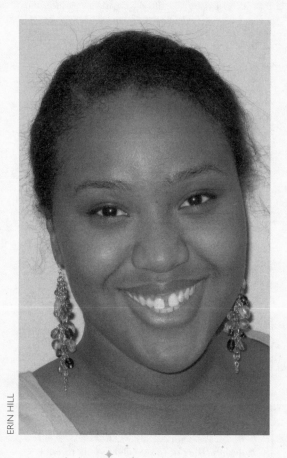

ERIN HILL

Guides to the Planet

When her acute myelogenous leukemia went into remission in 1998, Cambrey Thomas divided her life into two halves: sick and normal. Recently, as Thomas was celebrating ten years in remission, she realized that it would be far more fun to live one life—meshing all the experiences into one lifeline and accepting everything for what it is. When this native Detroiter is not working hard on her studies in college, drinking tea, or out seeing the world, she writes the blog "1-800-Cancer-Me," where she discusses the cultural and social implications of being a ten-year survivor (which includes everything from personal advocacy to comical misunderstandings to echocardiograms).

What it's really like to . . .
Have a Port Implanted and Get Chemotherapy for the First Time

by Heidi Schultz Adams

I think I can honestly say that it had never once occurred to me to think about what "chemo" really was before I was diagnosed with cancer. When my new oncologist said, "You'll be doing this chemotherapy protocol for twelve months," I didn't even know what to picture. Shots? Pills? Being tethered to an IV? I focused less on what it was and more on what I was afraid it would do to me; that I would be bald and bent over a toilet, retching, for the better part of the next year. But at that point, unable to walk and completely sleep-deprived from months of excruciating pain emanating from the newly discovered bone tumor in my left tibia, I was game for anything that might help.

Bingo on the IV, but not in my arm, as I had automatically pictured it. The first step toward receiving chemotherapy was to get a port-a-cath implanted in my chest—a device that would allow me to mainline the toxic chemicals that were supposed to save my life, so I wouldn't have to destroy the veins in my arms. They showed me a port, which looked like small, chunky, plastic Mickey Mouse ears filled with silicone, with a long tube snaking out of it.

About three weeks after the biopsy to my left ankle had confirmed a diagnosis of Ewing's sarcoma, my brother wheeled me into the hospital in the early morning for surgery to implant my port. I had just settled into my room when the phlebotomy tech came in to start prepping me for surgery. She looked at my arm and informed me that I had "good veins." I glowed at the praise. She deftly inserted an IV, and I went back to counting down the time until I would be wheeled into the operating room.

Finally, it was go-time. I laid back and made nervous small talk with the anesthesiologist as my bed was wheeled along the hospital corridors and into the operating room. It was very bright, and there were several people in scrubs and masks waiting for me. I don't remember much after that, although I have a vague recollection of saying something horribly inappropriate to the (handsome, male) anesthesiologist that I will to my dying day insist with great hope was just a dream.

Waking up in recovery was like being dragged out of a dark, cozy cave into a snowstorm, naked, with people yelling my name at me. I was freezing, nauseated, and the left side of my chest—right under my collarbone—hurt like hell. I just wanted to cover my ears, close my eyes, and crawl back into the cave.

I vaguely remember a machine being positioned over me and someone yelling "X-ray!"

at which point all medical personnel beat cheeks out of the room in no time flat. At the moment, fuzzy as I was, I remember finding this vaguely disturbing and slightly hilarious: that the several other moaning, retching patients lying on the beds around me were being involuntarily subjected to radiation, while all the able-bodied people managed to save themselves.

And then I was back in my room for the beginning of the first of many five-day stints in Hotel Baylor, Dallas, Texas. My chemotherapy protocol dictated an IV treatment every three weeks—blood counts allowing—alternating between five days of inpatient treatment and a one-day outpatient session. They had kindly accessed my port with a special hooked needle while I was under anesthesia, knowing that poking a needle through the swollen surgical site would hurt like hell. When I looked down, I saw tubing erupting directly out of my chest, flattened by a big, transparent, adhesive patch. The tubing was already hooked up to an IV, and I was receiving normal saline solution.

Later that day, the nurse came in to my room to "hang the bag" of chemo. There was a ritual to this that, I came to learn, did not vary. First, she put on a gown and gloves. She called another nurse into the room to double-check the label on the bag against my hospital wristband to make sure that these were really my drugs. She hung the bag onto my IV pole and connected it to the saline drip. A few button-punches to set the infusion rate of the pump, and that was that.

Sort of anticlimactic, really.

In anticipation of the projectile vomiting that was surely in my near future, I plotted my route to the bathroom, wondering how fast I could drag the IV pole without ripping the tubes out of my chest. But they had already prepped me with the antinausea wonder drug Zofran, and I never got past midlevel tummy turmoil on that particular stint.

I spent the next five days sleeping, waking, sleeping, and waking again as my IV tree slowly sprouted more and more bags and tubes. I don't remember too much, because I was availing myself freely of Ativan until I realized that I was losing large chunks of time to the black hole of chemical amnesia.

I didn't throw up. My hair didn't fall out overnight. It was no picnic in the park, but it wasn't devastatingly awful, either. And best of all, at the end of five days, I looked down at my left ankle and saw that it had magically deflated from being huge, red, swollen, and painful to looking—and feeling—just like its neighbor on the right. The nurse unhooked me from the IV, flushed my port with heparin so it wouldn't clot before the next time it was used, and gently withdrew the needle from my chest.

I reached up to touch the small lump under my skin. It was hard, and I could feel the outlines of the Mickey Mouse ears and the first couple of inches of tubing threading through my artery. I hopped out of bed, landing on both feet, and walked out of the room under my own power, pain-free for the first time in eight months. I thought about the next year stretching out interminably in front of me and said to myself, "Totally worth it."

Radiation

I had both my breasts removed four months ago. I didn't get new ones and have never worn my prosthesis. I went in for a post-chemo MUGA scan, and I was slated to go see my five-month-old niece afterward. To double-check and make sure I was not radioactive as a result of the MUGA scan—I turned out to be—I asked the technician if I was OK to hold a young baby.

Horrified, he looked at me and said, "Oh my God, you're not breastfeeding, are you?"

—Amanda

Evidently I am not holding my breath well enough. I think I am holding my breath, but it seems I am actually letting out a small amount of air. You hold your breath to pull your heart down away from the rays. Anyway, they say I will get better at it, and since I have it every day, five days a week for seven weeks, I have lots of opportunities to practice.

—Katie Jozwicki

I lost whatever modesty I had left. I felt like I was baring my chest for two different people—many of them men—every day. Quite an experience for someone who used to be really shy.

—Jess

Ah, radiation. In addition to (or instead of) the bull-in-a-china-shop M.O. of chemotherapy, radiation is a pinpointed ray of energy, either X-rays or gamma rays, targeted to wreak havoc on cancer cells in a very specific area.

Radiation therapy preys on the characteristic of cancer cells that makes them less able to restore themselves when damaged. The type of radiation you receive depends on your tumor and

> **Radiation therapy preys on the characteristic of cancer cells that makes them less able to restore themselves when damaged.**

its location. If you have skin cancer, for example, you won't undergo a high-energy beam because you don't require deep penetration beyond your skin. If your tumor is in your abdomen, on the other hand, you'll receive higher-energy radiation to reach it properly. No matter the energy level, you don't feel anything during a radiation therapy session.

So you sit, immobilized by various devices so your body is in the exact same position every time, and your tumor is zapped at very brief intervals—in most cases, less than five minutes, several times a week, for several weeks—and, whizbang, it takes out everything in its path. Your normal cells, better able to regenerate, will make it. The hope is that the cancer cells will not.

Internal radiation, or brachytherapy, is becoming more common in treating certain cancers. This type of radiation treatment surgically places a radiation source often referred to as "seeds" into or near a tumor for a particular (usually brief) period of time—the idea is that the more localized the radiation, the fewer healthy cells are affected.

You'll have a radiation oncologist to help plan and implement your therapy. He or she will explain your regimen and schedule, pinpoint the location of the zaps, and get after your tumor as though it's something stolen.

What it's really like to . . .
Obliterate Your Thyroid Cells with a Radioactive Pill

by Jessica Lindley

Six days after being diagnosed with papillary thyroid cancer at age thirty-two, I discovered I was two months pregnant. I postponed my treatments, and three months after my son's birth, I had a total thyroidectomy. Three months after my thyroidectomy, I began radioactive iodine therapy (RAI), which destroys the thyroid gland's tissue and cancer cells remaining from the thyroidectomy without harming your body's other tissue.

The radiation facility is physically and aesthetically freezing. It feels as if you're on a spaceship. I meet with the RAI doctor. The doctor has a thick accent. His voice and accent sound like Arnold Schwarzenegger. I can barely understand him. Dr. Schwarzenegger tells me I am going to take a pill that contains radioactive iodine, or I-131, which will kill any remaining thyroid cells as well as the cancer cells without (in theory) affecting the rest of my body, since the thyroid is the only part of your body that absorbs iodine. After I take the pill, all will be "good-good." He shows me a scan of my thyroid bed—it's now referred to as a thyroid bed since I have had my thyroid surgically removed—and points out swarms of little yellow dots. He tells me these are "bad-bad cells that must be exterminated."

Dr. Schwarzenegger then escorts me to a large lab and has me sit in an old metal school chair. It's freezing, and I am really happy that I do not have to wear a hospital gown and sit with my bare ass on the metal seat. Dr. Schwarzenegger leaves and says, "Someone will be with you." I was kinda hoping he would say, "I'll be back."

I am left alone in this stark-freezing-ass lab in jeans, a Ramones T-shirt, and flip-flops. Two men in spacesuits come in. Not kidding. They are in hooded respirator suits, and they are carrying what looks to be a very, very, very heavy box. The "spacemen" (with great effort) set the box on the counter. I now see that the box, which is the size of a small guitar amp or toaster oven, is solid lead. The spacemen ask me how my day is going and proceed to open the box. What exactly I am supposed to respond with is beyond me. "Awkward" and "freaky" come to mind, but I just mumble "fine." I am too intrigued with what is in the box and what exactly is going to happen to me, and if this is some weird experiment and where is the nearest exit. The spacemen pull a long cylinder out of the box. One of the spacemen holds the cylinder with his thick-gloved hands, and the other spaceman unscrews the cap. The entire time I can hear their breath, and their voices are like echoes. One of the men grabs some of the longest tongs I have ever seen, and at this point I am no longer intrigued—I am fucking terrified. He uses the tongs to pull out a small, yellow pill.

The other man hands me a cup of water and tells me to open my mouth and tilt my head back, and that they will now proceed to drop the pill down my throat. He also tells me to be sure and not let the pill touch any part of my mouth! I nod in submission. I am thinking, "What the fuck am I putting in my body and why does it matter if this radioactive pill that is going to irradiate all the 'bad-bad' cells in my body touches my tongue or teeth?!" So, the guy holding the pill with the very long tongs stands as far as he can from me and drops the pill down my throat. The other guy tells me to drink the water and they both pack up the box and they leave rather quickly. A speaker comes on and through static I hear Arnold Schwarzenegger's voice say, "You can come into my office now." I walk in his office, still freezing my ass off, and he waves a Geiger counter over me, pausing at my neck. The Geiger counter buzzes and beeps like crazy while Dr. Schwarzenegger mumbles "good-good." I am now officially radioactive. Dr. Schwarzenegger tells me to come back in five days and then, oh by the way, "No eating around or with other people, no sharing of food, no kissing, no extended physical touch, do not come in contact with pregnant women, and stay four to six feet away from children."

WTF?!?!? I have a six-month-old baby, and I eat out all the time! My husband and I look at each other and all I can think about is how fucking cold I am and that I cannot touch my son for five days.

We leave and begin calling friends and family to help out with taking care of our son. I feel exhausted. Since I have no thyroid, and since the goal is to get rid of all my remaining thyroid cells, I am not on any thyroid replacement drugs. I am extremely hypothyroid. I am fatigued, depressed, have severely dry skin, and have extreme trouble concentrating and remembering things—like words and names.

Did I say fatigued? The fatigue is nothing like I've ever felt. It is the feeling of being tired while you are sleeping and feeling as if you are physically caving in. My limbs feel heavy, and my mind is near comatose. I go home and sleep. I get up to pee and just happen to pee in the dark and my pee is glowing. Yes, I have glowing yellow pee! It looks as though I swallowed a yellow highlighter. I don't even want to think about what is going on inside my body. My husband makes a mistake and curls up next to me for a few minutes while I'm sleeping and his arm and leg become light red—as if they have been sunburned. We decide it is best for me to just curl up in the cave of my bedroom, sequester myself from the world, so I do not cause a radiation incident.

Over the next five days, I am alone. I wave to my son from across the room, have weird hot flashes, and have nausea and heartburn—gee, I wonder why? And I am continually fascinated by my glowing pee, which by the fifth day has lost a bit of its glow and becomes a dull yellow-brown. I try to read but cannot remember full sentences. I try to watch movies, but it's too hard to concentrate. When I eat, everything has a metallic taste to it. I feel that I'm losing my mind, that I'm physically falling apart, and that I'm totally alone while it's occurring. The radiation causes the metallic taste, glowing pee, nausea, heartburn, and hot flashes. The rest of my symptoms are from the hypothyroidism.

On the fifth day, I return to Dr. Schwarzenegger. He performs a scan and then shows me my thyroid bed, which now has just a few yellow dots. This is "good-good." Yippee! Fewer "bad-

bad" cells! Dr. Schwarzenegger scans my body with the Geiger counter, and it lazily hisses and intermittently beeps. The doc tells me everything is "good-good" and my radiation levels are optimum. I am free to go and can resume life as "normal." I need no more RAI treatments, and I can now begin my thyroid hormone-replacement therapy. I go home and toss all the radioactive linens and my "treatment" clothes, including my favorite Ramones T-shirt, into a burn pile—it was somewhat therapeutic.

Overall, the whole RAI process was surreal and maddening. The hardest part was having no real physical contact with people, especially when I was literally going through a mental and physical breakdown. I'm now cancer-free and have a balanced thyroid/endocrine system, but I still have a metallic taste in my mouth when I eat certain foods like cucumbers and melons. If I had to do it again, I wouldn't have worn my favorite T-shirt and I would've taken pictures of my pee!

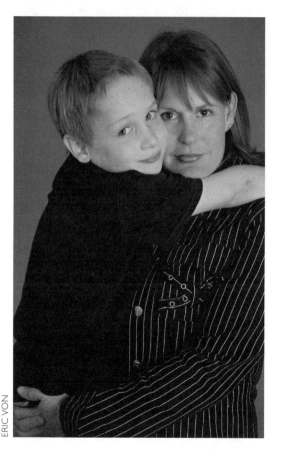

ERIC VON

Guides to the Planet

Jessica Lindley was diagnosed with papillary thyroid cancer at age thirty-two when she was two months pregnant. After having a healthy baby boy, she began her cancer treatment, which included a thyroidectomy, radiation treatment, and hormone therapy. After receiving treatment at M.D. Anderson, she became involved with Planet Cancer. Jessica lives in Austin, Texas, with her very healthy son. She is currently undergoing treatment for recurring, well-differentiated thyroid cancer. Laughter being the best medicine, you can usually find Jessica at some Austin coffee shop laughing—mostly, she says, at herself. She enjoys fine dining, music, and moonlit walks along the beach.

Some specific types of specialized radiation:

Tomotherapy delivers precise, targeted doses of radiation throughout a tumor by using special software that allows CT scans to document a tumor in 3-D. This technology also cuts down on the radiation that hits healthy tissue around the tumor.

Proton Beam Therapy uses a beam of protons instead of X-rays to radiate tumors. The unique characteristic of protons is that when they hit the tumor, they give up the ghost—along with most of their energy. Because of this, they don't have an "exit dose" after they travel through the tumor, so there's less impact on healthy surrounding tissue, allowing greater doses to be given with fewer side effects.

Gamma Knife Surgery. No, we didn't put this in the wrong section. The gamma knife uses radiation for a single session of "stereotactic radiosurgery," which, though it sounds as if it could be, is not an album put out by a Wu-Tang splinter group. It doesn't remove the tumor but basically deactivates it to prevent further growth. After extensive preplanning, intense, highly focused beams of radiation hit a 3-D target with extreme precision—to a fraction of a millimeter. A gamma knife session may last a few minutes or hours, depending on dose, size, and shape of the target (usually less than four centimeters in size). The gamma knife is so precise that it can blast a tumor while, for the most part, sparing the surrounding tissue. This is particularly important when you're going after something unwanted in, for example, the brain or spine.

> More than half of all those who undergo cancer treatment will receive some form of radiation therapy.

What it's really like to . . .
Receive Brain Radiation

by Joshua Lipschutz

Before any radiation was administered, there was a planning meeting that lasted an hour or two. They created a mold for a mask to hold my head in the same position each time my brain was radiated. They put small tattoos on my head and neck to help position my head for perfect alignment. Once the mold was created, they took me into the room where the radiation happened.

The room was big and open, and it had a medical table in the middle. Above the table was a machine that looked like a huge telescope. This machine took pictures and beamed radiation. The radiation technician positioned me and left the room, closing what appeared to be a two-foot-thick door behind him. At that point, the table rotated 360 degrees and went up and down while the machine remained stationary throughout the radiation administration.

Several scans were performed at the onset to ensure everything was in position. After about another hour, I was ready. I went home with a moderate amount of anxiety. Was it going to be painful? Were there going to be long-term effects? Was it even going to work?

The treatment itself was painless. It was inconvenient going five days a week for six weeks, but after getting into a routine, it became easier.

As treatment progressed, I experienced some unpleasant side effects: About two or three weeks into radiation, I began to lose my hair in patches, particularly in the area that was being radiated. The skin on my scalp became dry and irritated, almost like sunburn. I also became fatigued, often needing a midafternoon nap. This became much worse toward the end of radiation, when I was tired all the time.

I experienced terrible headaches at times. These were not always responsive to medication. Probably the worst part of it all was the Decadron, a steroid used to help with swelling in the brain. The Decadron made me ravenous. My appetite could not be satisfied. So, I gained a lot of weight and I was really tired—not a great combination. Every time they tried to wean me off Decadron, my headaches worsened.

In all, the six weeks went by rather quickly. Radiation to the brain is utterly painless—a little unnerving, but painless. It's the drugs and side effects that suck.

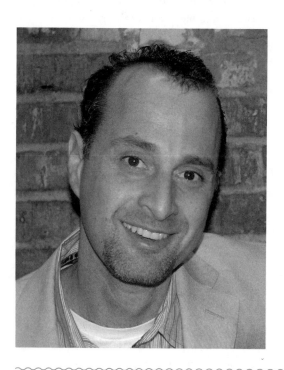

Guides to the Planet

Joshua Lipschutz was diagnosed with Grade II astrocytoma, a tumor in the left occipital region of his brain, in 1992, at age twenty-one. The tumor was removed in December 1992. In October 2006, Josh was diagnosed with Grade III astrocytoma: a tumor in the left occipital region that had spread to the corpus callosum. Fourteen years after his first surgery, he underwent another brain operation. He then had six weeks of brain radiation along with ongoing (thirty-five+) cycles of chemotherapy.

Josh plays tennis, sails, and travels as much as possible.

Surgery

I'm kind of freaking out right now. I really want to cancel my surgery and just get on with life like nothing happened. I mean, don't want to miss out on the fun this summer. But hey, it's an experience, and what doesn't kill me makes me stronger, right? So off I will go for another surgery.

—TINLUNCHBOX

When the docs decide it's time to give certain of your malfunctioning body parts the boot, you'll be staring down the barrel of surgery. Hours of presurgery prep work include blood draws, a list of every medication you've ever even held, and a history of every previous surgery/diagnosis/headache/menstrual period/nasty thought you've ever had. Come prepared with a list of these things to make the trip smoother.

In your pre-op visit, you'll also get a chance to meet with an anesthesiologist (likely not the one who'll be actually administering your anesthesia the day of). If you are going to be intubated for surgery, they'll tell you and give you the opportunity to request a small-sized tube. (Do it.) You can also request specific antinausea meds for pre- and post-surgery, like a scopolamine patch (commonly used to prevent motion sickness).

The day of surgery, you'll check in if you aren't already an inpatient, and go to the pre-op area. Leave contact lenses and valuable jewelry at home. Come with a hair tie if you have long hair (or any hair). You'll be dressed in a gown, sexy compression socks, and a hair net straight from lunch lady land. Your surgeon should come in to talk to you and your family members, giving you all a brief description of the day's events and what to expect.

> Compression socks, or compression stockings, or, for the hard core, "thrombo-embolic deterrent stockings" are specially designed footwear—super-opaque, super-thick white knee-highs with the toes cut out, like a sock puppet depicting an Arctic explorer—that lower the risk of getting blood clots in your legs during surgery or prolonged bed rest. They're designed to apply effective pressure in the right places—i.e., more on your feet than your ankles.

What should you expect? Expect to request lots of blankets, because it gets cold in pre-op with only a cotton gown. Expect to have a catheter inserted into your vein for the anesthesiologist during surgery. Expect a parade of nurses, anesthesia assistants, and the like to be coming in and out, taking your blood pressure and your vital signs and telling you not to worry.

After they've pre-opped you to their hearts' content, you'll have a syringe of midazolam, or Versed ("vitamin V" in hospital slang) pushed into your catheter, and you won't remember a darn thing from there on out. Versed doesn't physically block any pain, but it keeps you from laying down any short-term memories, so you won't remember being wheeled from pre-op into the surgery room. You won't remember saying good-bye to your family members or calling the surgeon "Big Boy" as he pats your hand and asks after your well-being. You won't remember being hoisted onto the operating table or the bright lights bearing down on you. You'll be fully awake, but you won't remember any of this. And that's for the best.

You'll remember waking up, hours later, in the recovery room, with your family and a cup of flat ginger ale by your side. You'll remember puking into a pink plastic kidney bean-shaped bowl. You'll remember not being allowed to leave the hospital until you pee—if you're in overnight, you'll also have to produce some poop. And you'll certainly remember being constipated for days, because anesthesia stops you up. (No pre-op info includes that factoid.)

No matter what you forget, don't forget to have family and friends with you post-operatively. They can talk to the surgeons about the results of the surgery, because otherwise you won't remember a word that was said.

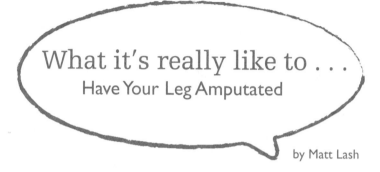

What it's really like to . . .
Have Your Leg Amputated

by Matt Lash

It sucks. I mean, how else should I put it? It sucks to have your leg amputated. And I challenge anyone to a game of "Stand on One Leg" who answers this question with "It's pretty cool." New questions pop into your mind after you have your amputation, ones you'd never think of before: How long will it take for me to pass through airport security? Should I fake limp out of my car when I park in a handicap space so people think I'm justified for parking so close? When do I tell this cute girl that when she plays footsie with me, I might not feel it? Lots of new questions. So no, it's not cool.

All that being said, it's pretty freaking cool to have your leg amputated. I know I'm contradicting myself, but who cares? I have cancer and can do what I want. (That response usually wins every argument; be sure to use it if necessary.)

I get to the hospital on "cutting day" at 5 a.m., and the doctors mark an "X" on the correct leg.

They write on the other leg, "Do not cut." I give Mommy and Daddy and Girlfriend kisses and exchange a crying moment before they give me the great drugs and loop me up.

I wake up with a huge cast on, with a metal rod and a plastic foot extending from the cast, but I don't really care because I'm so stoned from the painkillers that I think Jesus is in my room collecting cans (I swear). With help from parents and rehabbing, I reteach myself how to walk in about two months. It hurts, but your leg heals. I reteach myself how to climb steps, jog, and dance. My leg sends me pain signals called phantom pain, which is basically your brain reworking its wires to realize there's no leg anymore. This pain is good, because it helps you keep balance, since you know where your leg should be. I begin to do thirty minutes on the elliptical workout machine. I suck at running long distances, but I always sucked.

I travel to Europe for two weeks with buddies. I take my leg off in the middle of a huge parade in Germany and wave it around amid hundreds of onlookers. A friendly Australian steals my leg one

> **My tour guide tells me I can stay at the bottom of Mount Masada if I don't think I can make it up. I beat him to the top.**

night while we're all getting drunk and eventually passes out with it in his arms. I graduate in five years, three of them involving surgeries and chemo. I walk across the stage. I live in Spain for a study abroad program in law school. I use an old pizza box as padding for my leg because I dance literally all night in San Sebastián. I see the sun set and rise too many times to count on the beaches of Santander. I travel to Israel. I meet the most beautiful women in the world there and get shot down by all of them! My tour guide tells me I can stay at the bottom of Mount Masada if I don't think I can make it up. I beat him to the top. I also climb a mountain overlooking Jordan and Syria. I ride a camel.

I graduate from law school. I stand as best man to watch my brother marry his beautiful bride. I get to hold my new baby niece, Ella, and kiss her chubby face when she is born. She later pees on my shirt.

So, yes, it's also pretty freaking cool.

Guides to the Planet

Matt Lash was diagnosed with Ewing's sarcoma at age twenty. He's pictured here with his niece, Ella, at age twenty-seven. Matt passed away before this book was completed; we're proud that his contribution, witty and soulful, is here so that readers can know him.

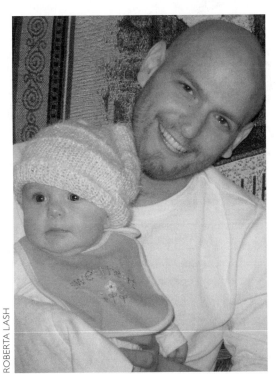

ROBERTA LASH

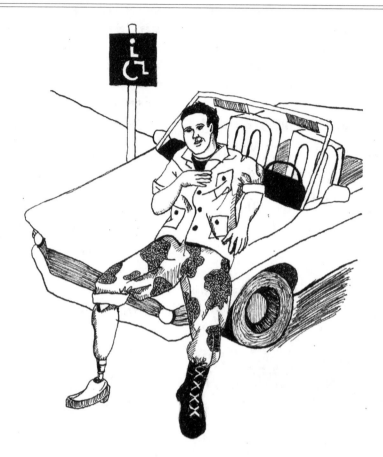

Top 10 Benefits of a Prosthetic Limb

10. It ups your street cred when you lie about how you were "in the shit."

9. You kick ass at that hold-your-hand-over-the-flame game.

8. Buying shoes. Easy for you, confusing for them.

7. You can freak out roller-coaster technicians by "losing a limb" during the ride and playing air guitar with it when you're done.

6. Sunburn—never a worry.

5. If you have the money, in a flourish of individualism, you can leave limbs around like calling cards.

4. They render unnecessary those unsightly and cluttering scratching posts for your cats.

3. Clear the kids out of the pool by humming the theme from *Jaws* while the limb gently floats by.

2. Three words: grease pencil tattoos.

1. Great parking.

Scars

I have an eight-inch vertical scar on my abdomen, and I've told people I got stabbed. Which is not technically untrue.

—Rebecca

When treatment is over, many physical aspects of cancer disappear. Hair grows back, body weight normalizes, taste and smell return. What remain, however, are small (or, too often, ginormous) reminders of the cancer experience: scars.

Scars are left from a variety of operations necessary for treatment, and some chemotherapy and radiation treatments leave permanent ones. Survivors can often be spotted wearing small, subclavian badges of honor left over from central lines or port-a-caths. Bleomycin, a commonly used chemotherapeutic agent, often scars its recipients inside and out, leaving trademark tiger stripes of hyperpigmentation on the skin and fibrous scar tissue in the lungs. Then there are biopsy scars and, usually more dramatic, the surgical leftovers of limb salvages—surgery that removes bone cancer or a soft-tissue sarcoma while sparing the affected limb—which can span an entire leg or arm. Scalp scars from brain surgery are also telling, as hair never grows over an incision site.

Although cancer leaves much to be desired aesthetically, most survivors don't seem to be deterred by the remnants of their journey. They wear their scars with pride, as symbols of strength and courage that will never fade away.

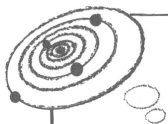

Dispatches from the Planet

I had to have a big chunk of my upper right leg taken out for melanoma treatment before taking my high school students to Costa Rica. I did not want to tell them about the cancer until we got back from the trip. One of my fellow teachers told the students that I had been out for a week because I had flown to Costa Rica early and had been bitten by a large shark. He told them not to ask me about it because I did not want them to be scared, and it was too late for them to drop out of the trip. The students believed the whole story! They now know the truth but still ask how my numerous shark bites are healing.

—Kris

I work retail, and sometimes my port scar shows. Most of the people that comment are other people who know what the scar is because they have one too! It's kind of cool to talk to other people about it. Makes ya not feel so alone!

—red85

How to Cover Up Your Scars

We asked Lori Ovitz, the most accomplished stylist-slash-magician on Planet Cancer, to teach us how to cover up scars. Read on if you want to learn how to make your scar(s) disappear, courtesy of a master. (Lori is a professional makeup artist in Chicago; she's worked with top models and celebrities.) These tips come to us courtesy of Lori from her book, *Facing the Mirror with Cancer.*

If you want to cover up your scar(s), you need to use camouflage, heavy-duty concealer designed for things like scars and tattoos. Unlike other types of makeup, camouflage covers a specific spot. It can be used on other parts of the body and doesn't have to be restricted to the face. (And it doesn't *remove* the scar—camouflage derives from the French word for "disguise," not "sandblaster.") Camouflage doesn't come in as many colors as foundation, but try to get your camouflage to be the same tone as your foundation (and your skin tone). "If you're using the right product," Lori says, "you shouldn't need any colors."

The Technique:

1. Use your finger, a sponge, or a concealer brush, depending on the size of the area where you are applying camouflage.

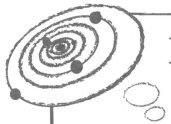

Dispatches from the Planet

I've had quite a few questions on my port scars lately (I'm a fan of low-cut shirts). I find if I say something ridiculous, like that I was harpooned, and get a guy to give me the "you're shitting me" look, I can de-escalate the story to a real snoozer—it was just cancer. This seems to break the ice. People follow up with questions. Questions are good. I'm not saying they want to date me, but at least they're talking and not avoiding eye contact.

—KayCee

After I had surgery to remove two large tumors from my liver, I ended up with a huge scar that looks like the peace sign or the Mercedes-Benz logo. The scar covers my whole stomach. Most people thought I would never wear a bikini again, but how wrong they were! I am very proud of my trophy! In the beginning I was a little self-conscious, but now, after five years, my belly is once again my favorite part of my body. It reminds me of how lucky I am.

—Danielle Duran Baron

2. Apply camouflage with a little dab, as follows:

- Gently pat the camouflage onto the area you want to cover.

- Press it on. No rubbing or smearing. We're pressing and patting here!

- Continue to press-pat, press-pat. The motion is kind of a "hopalong."

- Always remember to be gentle. Tap softly to blend it in. Do not rub or smear.

3. Use the press-pat technique until the camouflage is totally blended in with your skin. This technique is important in getting the thick camouflage to effectively cover an area without clumping or appearing too light or too dark. If you press-pat, you will zero in on the area you want to conceal. If you rub it in, the camouflage will spread out over a much wider area.

If you use foundation, it goes on after the camouflage. (*Note:* You don't have to use foundation to do this scar-covering technique.)

Another tip from Lori: "A lot of time people want to add tons of makeup. No, no, no!" she says. "You'll look like a clown."

Top 10 Responses to Nosy Questions about Scars

10. Never go to Mother's Tattoo Parlor when you're high.

9. You think that's bad, you should see the exit wound.

8. I self-mutilate. Don't you?

7. Those damn flesh-eating bacteria are spreading. Slowly, but surely.

6. That's where the government put the chip to track my movements.

5. It's the only way to smuggle drugs these days.

4. What scar? What are you talking about? Oh my God! That's **huge!**

3. I had to sell organs to get off the street.

2. I should have listened when Mom said not to scratch that mosquito bite.

1. That's where my Siamese twin was attached.

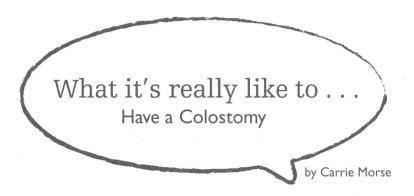

What it's really like to . . .
Have a Colostomy

by Carrie Morse

"I'm 99 percent sure it's cancer. We won't know for sure until the biopsy comes back. But you'll most likely have chemo and radiation and then surgery where they'll remove your rectum and you'll have a permanent colostomy. . . . " The doctor who had just shoved things up my ass kept talking after that, but *colostomy* was the last word I heard. When he finished talking, I asked what that meant, and he said I'd have a colostomy bag. Then he said, "Not to worry. The appliances are much better than they used to be."

Appliances? What the hell? I was picturing a dishwasher or a stove hanging off my belly. Or a rolling suitcase full of shit. That did not sound appealing.

I did everything I could to find out what it was like to have a colostomy before they cut my bunghole out. There are some awesome message boards out there. The United Ostomy Associations of America (UOAA) boards were really helpful in learning about all the different kinds of appliances. One piece, two piece, closed bag, bag with clip—there are lots of different "systems" out there. I learned that the wafer is the part that sticks to your skin and sometimes the bag is attached to the wafer—a one piece. And sometimes the bag snaps onto the wafer—that's a two-piece. Some bags are open at the bottom

and are held closed with a clip and you empty them when they're full. Then there are the closed bags that get tossed out when they're full. Even with gaining all this information beforehand, I don't think anything can truly prepare you for what it's really like to shit in a bag that hangs off your stomach.

My experience has been difficult. I had a terrible time finding a bag and wafer that worked. They kept lifting and I'd end up with stool underneath the wafer and my skin got really irritated. Anyone who has an ostomy of any kind knows that keeping your parastomal skin clean, dry, and in good condition is the most important thing to having a "good ostomy experience." Good ostomy experience? I want to smack people who say that since none of them actually have colostomies.

After a lot of trial and error, I eventually went to the simplest system possible, and it works pretty well. Dot, the stoma nurse at Georgetown Hospital, was amazing in helping me find something that worked. Stoma nurses are angels. They know the tricks of the trade—not things you'll find in any packaging or instructions from the ostomy supply manufacturers. It's stuff you learn from other ostomates and stoma nurses.

I use a two-piece closed-bag system, and I change my wafer daily. I take the wafer off before

I shower and I shower naked. It's the only time I am truly naked. It's such a nice feeling. I shit all over my shower regularly, but it doesn't bug me

> Even with gaining all this information beforehand, I don't think anything can truly prepare you for what it's really like to shit in a bag that hangs off your stomach.

anymore. I shit on my floor too. Sometimes my stoma expels and I don't realize it or I can't stop it in time and, plop—it's on the floor. It doesn't freak me out as I thought it would. It's more of a nuisance than anything else as I usually have to spend twenty to thirty minutes cleaning up after it happens and I end up late if I am going somewhere. Most of the time I laugh. But some days I lose it and loudly say something like, "Are you fucking kidding me?!" When that happens, my dog looks at me like "What'd I do?" It's funny that I am the one pooping on the floor, not him! I have also shit on my dog. He was lying on the bathroom rug once when my stoma let loose and he was in the line of fire. Such is life with a stoma.

My stoma was really noisy for the first several months. It released gas at very inopportune moments. Oddly enough, that was no big deal. I told my coworkers to expect it to make noise during staff meetings, and my friends all knew about it. It still makes noise, but I can kind of tell when it's gonna fart and I can press my hand on it. If it goes off, I just say, "'scuse me." The good

thing is, I can rip a massive fart and no one can smell it!

It took a while for my stoma to "normalize" since I started adjuvant chemo within a month after surgery, and that made me shit with no regularity. Sometimes I'd have to change my bag five times a day and sometimes I'd go through a whole day without changing it. Once things started normalizing, I had to have another surgery to repair a ventral hernia and a stomal hernia, and things got all mucked up again. My colon takes a long time to wake up after surgery.

Despite crazy crapping habits, I started doing "normal" things as soon as I could. Swimming, for example: I was in the pool within five weeks of my surgery. That was easier than I thought it'd be, and as a sun worshipper and former swimming teacher—the pool was a sanctuary while I was recovering.

Having a colostomy has forced me to plan ahead more than I used to. I feel as if I can't be as spontaneous as I used to be. I always need to know where the bathroom is and if there will be a bathroom. I hope someday that will change, but I've had my stoma for less than two years and I am still nervous sometimes. I always have

---

Ostomies and stomas aren't the same: According to the United Ostomy Associations of America, an **ostomy** is an opening in the body created via surgery for the discharge of wastes; a **stoma** is "the actual end of the ureter or small or large bowel" that protrudes through the abdominal wall. Learn more from their site: www.uoaa.org. *Note:* "Stoma" is the Greek word for "mouth."

at least five extra bags with me and a wafer and everything I'd need to change my whole rig if I have to. I've had to do that three times. Twice in the bathroom at work and once in an airport bathroom. Man did I stink up the airport bathroom!!

And that's one more thing—colostomies are smelly. Really, really smelly. Shit comes out and it's right there. But it's amazing how I've become used to it. Shit doesn't gross me out at all. More normal things, like someone else's half-eaten food on a plate—disgusting. Tons and tons of shit—not so much.

Sometimes I feel as though people expect me to not care about the stoma since I'm alive and that's the most important thing. And hopefully I'll get there someday. But for now I am still trying to find a new normal and get used to what it's really like to have a stoma, since it's really there and will be there forever. *C'est la guerre.*

Guides to the Planet

Carrie Morse lives in Washington, D.C., with her ferocious dog/four-legged angel, Deke. On December 23, 2006, at age thirty-four, she was diagnosed with rectal cancer. In January 2007 she began two months of chemo along with thirty radiation treatments that were utter torture. Then she had the surgery that, she says, "stole my bunghole and gave me a permanent colostomy."

When she's not roaming the halls of Georgetown Hospital, she can be found at almost every home Washington Capitals hockey game. In the months between hockey seasons, she spends as much time as possible at her favorite place in the world: her family's cottage in Northern Michigan. In March 2009 she was diagnosed with follicular

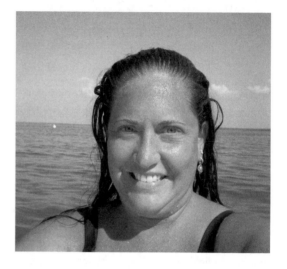

lymphoma, a form of non-Hodgkin's B-cell lymphoma. Follicular lymphoma is not curable, so, she says, "My Planet Cancer passport is going to get some more stamps in the future." She recently celebrated her thirty-seventh birthday by taking trapeze lessons.

Transplants

As the days and weeks went by, I swear those four walls were closing in! And when you get to leave your room, that lovely IV pole has to come along. I wasn't allowed to leave the transplant area at first, so I would walk up and down the same hallway over and over and over again. I was in the hospital for thirty-five days during my transplant.

—LAUREN

A transplant replaces your crappy, depleted immune system with one that's newer and better. It's a sort of rescue after high-dose chemotherapy, which beats your immune system down to a point at which screaming "Uncle!" would be an achievement. Transplants are most commonly used for cancers that affect your blood and lymph systems, such as leukemia, lymphoma, myeloma, and melanoma.

There are two primary types of stem cell transplants: **Autologous SCTs** use your own blood; **allogeneic** procedures use stem cells from a donor (sibling, parent, or perfect stranger). A

> How to bathe with drains from breast surgery: Surgical drains (tubes used to remove pus, blood, etc., from a wound caused by surgery) have safety pins to pin them to your gown so they don't hang loose. After my last breast surgery, I took an old swimsuit and cut the neckline out of the rest of the suit. I hung the neckline around my neck and pinned my drains to it—so I had a strip of material that was fine to get wet hanging around my neck to stabilize the drains.

> ### Bone Marrow Transplant or Stem Cell Transplant?
>
> The magic cells that have the ability to regrow an entire blood-making/immune system are called hematopoietic stem cells, and they normally live in people's bone marrow. If you get them by taking out bone marrow in the operating room, it's called a **bone marrow transplant** (BMT). If you collect them through *apheresis* (filtering blood on a dialysis-like machine), it's called a **peripheral blood stem cell transplant** (PBSCT, or SCT for short). If you get them from umbilical cord blood, it's called a **cord blood transplant,** and so on. The most correct term to describe any of these is *hematopoietic stem cell transplant* (HSCT). Many, however, still simply say BMT to mean any and all of these.

third, **syngeneic,** uses stem cells from an identical twin and is less common for obvious reasons.

Many things happen before the transplant. Chemotherapy reduces or eliminates the cancer. Bone marrow stimulants such as Neupogen and Neulasta shots increase cell counts. And there's a process called apheresis. During apheresis, the stem cells are sucked from the blood, sealed tight, frozen, and stored while awaiting transplant. When all the preparations are complete and your old immune system is out of commission, the new cells are put back into your body intravenously.

Side effects from the pre-transplant preparations and the transplant itself may include but are not limited to nausea, vomiting, diarrhea, constipation, hair loss, mouth sores, infections, anemia, fatigue, organ failure, and even secondary cancers. Sounds fun, right?

In donor transplants, graft-versus-host disease, or GVHD, is another potential side effect. GVHD is a war between the donor cells and your body, and the fallout can range from mild to quite serious.

> When transplants are discussed, you'll start to hear the term "perfect match." In an allogeneic transplant, the donor marrow must match six out of six "markers" to be a perfect match. These markers are human leukocyte antigens (HLAs), which are found on white blood cells. They help assess the compatibility of your immune system with your donor's. Half your markers come from each parent, so each sibling has a one-in-four chance of matching. Less than half of us have a sibling who matches, so there's a national registry of more than five million volunteer donors.

During and after the transplant, isolation may be necessary to give the new immune system a chance to develop. Fear not: Only the most compromised patients are confined to a bubble. Generally, inpatient care is all that is required to separate you from all those bastards who won't cover their mouths when they cough.

A transplant is not a simple process. That's why arming yourself with as much information as possible will increase your chances of making it through one alive. The good news is that, through the help of clinical trials and research, tremendous progress is being made in reducing most side effects from transplants and increasing not only your chance of living but also living without cancer.

What it's really like to . . .
Have a Stem Cell Transplant

by Kyle Steuck

It was May 13, and I smelled like creamed corn. Or garlic or fish or something, depending on whom you asked. I smelled the preservative chemical, DMSO or some other medical acronym, for only a few hours. Everyone else smelled it for days. It had kept my stem cells, or at least the few million sucked and spun from my blood by the apheresis machine, from being destroyed in the freezers. Those little frozen bits of me, carrying the power to make any

of the blood cells I needed, had been on ice for a month while the rest of me was battered by total-body irradiation and high-dose chemotherapy.

My doctor was a little too excited at the beginning of the process: "Young guy like you? We can really beat the crap out of you." Apparently beating the crap out of me was going to make me better. But first, it was definitely going to make me worse. A week of high-dose chemo and radiation wiped out my bone marrow, and I survived on a regular diet of transfusions and isolation from as many bugs as could be kept away. Anytime I came home, the houseplants were taken outside, and I wore a mask in public. On day three post-transplant, I spiked a fever due to an unspecific infection and landed in the hospital for the next eight days until my white blood cell count began to rise.

In the hospital, they watched everything that came into or left my body. The daily weighings came at 5 a.m., and the schedule for dozens of meds filled the rest of the day. The neutropenic diet (see "Immunosuppression" in chapter 4) meant no uncooked fruit or vegetables and an even blander version of the hospital bland diet (yes, it's possible to make hospital food taste worse). Eventually, the morphine and Ativan prevented me from remembering it all, and the days blurred together. I spoke to people who weren't really there and had to turn off a basketball game once because I couldn't keep track of who was playing long enough for the players to inbound the ball. I struggled out of bed to walk two or three laps down the short

hallway and spent several days in too much pain to speak or eat.

And then, slowly, my system recovered. The reawakened stem cells set up shop in my bone marrow and started on their to-do list: red cells, then platelets, then white cells. As the counts rose, the pill counts dropped and I felt better. Five days into the hospital stay, day eight, I slurped on a melted orange popsicle, then ate some soggy Cheerios, working my way toward more and more solid food. Following my bone marrow's lead, the rest of my battered body was putting itself back together. On May 24, day eleven, I left the hospital for good.

For another three weeks, I was in the clinic three times a week, ending on June 13, a month post-transplant. I spent the summer recovering. I left the mask behind, started eating more and more varied foods. I walked more, visited the hospital where I was originally diagnosed, made plans to return to college in the fall. More than three months later, one hundred days after my stem cells returned to my body, I had my last appointment with the transplant team. A few weeks after that, I was back in school. I had returned.

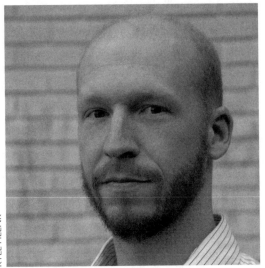

KYLE HEENK

Guides to the Planet

Kyle Steuck was diagnosed with Stage IV Hodgkin's at age nineteen. He was treated with a variety of therapies, including an autologous stem cell transplant. During the SCT, he swore he'd never sit on a bike seat again but is now an avid cyclist. After finishing treatment, he completed his degree and now lives in Seattle, where he practices structural engineering.

Other Treatments

Following are some additional treatment techniques that you might come across, new and beyond the standard methods. We're getting pretty advanced.

Hormone Therapy

Some cancers need specific hormones for their cells to keep growing. Hormone therapy works in a few different ways: either by stopping production of a specific hormone needed by the cancer, blocking a tumor's ability to use a hormone, or—the Trojan horse method—sneaking in a similar hormone that doesn't work, which means the cancer cells won't grow. Hormone therapy can be used either as a treatment for hormone-sensitive cancers or as an adjuvant treatment to prevent tumors from coming back after they're removed.

Because this therapy directly affects how your body processes and produces hormones, side effects can range from male and female hot flashes to enlarged breasts in men (Oh yes: See "What It's Really Like to . . . Grow Moobies, or Man Boobs" in chapter 4) and weight gain in women.

Immunotherapy

The idea behind immunotherapy is that we can rev up the body's immune system, turbocharging our own natural defenses to better recognize and fight cancer when it shows up. Immunotherapy includes biological response modifiers (BRM), such as interferons and interleukins, and tumor vaccines, which are still largely in the research phase.

Steroids

Many chemotherapy treatments complement whatever drugs you're getting with a ration of steroids. Steroids do one of two things: reduce swelling or lessen sickness. Often, tumors or radiation will cause swelling in surrounding tissue, and steroids temper this swelling. (Patients with brain cancer often take dexamethasone, a steroid, to reduce swelling of the brain tissue surrounding a tumor, and thus lessen headache pain.) Steroids given to reduce sickness are taken in much smaller doses. Steroids are the chief culprit of 'roid rage, which you can read about in chapter 4.

The Future:

Gene Therapy, Targeted Therapy

It's the understatement of the year to say that your body is complex. It's made of different tissues and organs formed by cells, which are made of even smaller components, including proteins. Your proteins are encoded by about twenty-five thousand genes that contain your genetic code. Your cells must grow and divide in exquisite coordination to function properly: Every time a cell division occurs, the genetic code of parental cells must be copied exactly and passed to resulting cells. Each individual's genetic code has nearly three billion characters!

A persistent alteration within these three billion characters is a mutation. Mutations can either be inherited from our parents or acquired over the course of our lives from environmental factors, such as chemical exposure or a bad habit like drinking Freon. Mutations within a variety of genes can trigger the onset of cancer, characterized by cells that grow out of control, brakes off and hammer down. The complicated nature of cell division is why there's no single "magic bullet" cure for cancer.

A goal of current cancer research is to significantly increase the effectiveness of treatment while diminishing the side effects. By better understanding how certain genetic changes correspond to specific disease states, we will be able to break down "cancer" into increasingly specific subgroups and be able to treat it better.

So what about that "magic bullet" (or, perhaps more accurately, "bullets")? A better understanding of the genetic identifications of various cancers will increasingly yield more precise weapons to be used against them, targeting the cancer cells and leaving your other cells alone. Unlike chemotherapy, which indiscriminately attacks both cancer cells and many of your body's normal cells, biologic agents in gene therapy strengthen your immune system to help it fight cancer cells.

The relatively new realm of biologic therapies (such as antibody-, vaccine-, cytokine-, and gene-based approaches) is certainly exciting. (Can't you just *feel* it?!) Ongoing and future research will assist in better detection and more powerful means of diagnosis and prognosis, as well as improved therapy under the laudable and desirable umbrella of more personalized medicine.

Clinical Trials

A plus for trials is that ideally a group of smart individuals have decided on an investigational therapy that is expected to have a good chance of being better than the standard practice. And if it wasn't for clinical trials, then cancer treatment wouldn't have improved to what it is now and will never be any better.

—LUKE

In the quest for equal cancer treatment for all, the clinical trial represents one of the greatest hurdles that young adults have to overcome. Suffice it to say that if you're age fifteen to thirty-nine, nobody's beating your door down to participate in a clinical trial: As the statistical outlier between pediatric and geriatric, you're not really in the sweet spot for a trial. Nobody is proactively recruiting you to trials, and you and your young adult peers aren't typically treated at academic centers, where the trials take place. Children are mainstays in clinical trials, as are older adults, but adolescents and young adults are largely left in the dust. This becomes particularly important when you consider research showing that age-dependent survival may be linked to rates of participation in and availability of clinical trials. The argument goes: Young adults aren't represented in clinical trials as well as their older and younger counterparts are; ergo, improvement in their survival rates hasn't kept pace, either.

Before we address this disparity, let's clear up exactly what clinical trials are (and aren't: For some frighteningly wrong depictions of clini-

> The risks involved in clinical trials mostly mirror the inherent risks of any treatment for a life-threatening illness.

cal trials on the TV series *Grey's Anatomy*, see "Popular Culture's Finest Misrepresentations of Young Adult Cancer" in chapter 4). First and most important, clinical trials aren't any more dangerous than normal cancer treatment. The risks involved in clinical trials mostly mirror the inherent risks of any treatment for a life-threatening illness. In fact, given the strict guidelines required in clinical trials to ensure consistent and accurate data, you may actually be more closely monitored and supported when you're on a trial. Also, patients in clinical trials are making a valuable contribution to cancer research, so you're helping yourself and the Planet at the same time. (See the list in the following section for more myth busting.)

Lots of reasons are tossed around to explain low participation by adolescents and young adults in clinical trials, including but probably not limited to limited eligibility, infrequent referrals from clinicians and doctors, fewer young adults treated at academic centers, and common mis-

understandings about clinical trial treatment options. Advocacy groups are making progress to incorporate more young adults in clinical trials, and the latest data points to progress being made. That said, we have a long way to go.

What can you do? Beat the drum loudly. Go after as much information as you can about trials you may qualify for, and talk with your doctors to make an informed decision.

Phases of Clinical Trials

Clinical trials occur in phases, each with a different goal. If there is a generally accepted

---

Top 10 Myths about Cancer Clinical Trials

The following list clears up some of the many misconceptions about clinical trials. It was put together by the Coalition of Cancer Cooperative Groups (CCCG), a nonprofit providing education and services to help understand cancer clinical trials as a treatment option. Check out the coalition online: www.CancerTrialsHelp.org.

1. **The doctor knows best. He or she will say whether I should participate.**

   Fact: Only you can decide whether to take part in a clinical trial. The role of your doctor and the rest of the care team is to provide you balanced information about the risks and benefits of participation in the trial you're interested in.

2. **Cancer clinical trial patients are given sugar pills.**

   Fact: Patients who join clinical trials are given the best treatment available or the chance to receive a new treatment being considered. Sugar pills (also called placebos) are rarely used in cancer clinical trials and are never used in place of treatment. What's more, these trials are

carefully monitored, so if a problem arises, the trial can be altered or stopped.

3. **Patients in clinical trials are treated like guinea pigs.**

   Fact: Of the 5,900 cancer patients surveyed by CCCG, virtually every clinical trial participant said that he or she was treated with dignity and respect, that the quality of care was "good" or "excellent," and that the overall experience was positive.

4. **Clinical trials are too risky.**

   Fact: Most clinical trials aren't any more risky than normal treatment. Moreover, in clinical trials, patients are watched more closely by their doctor and other members of their medical team.

5. **Health insurance will not cover the costs of a clinical trial.**

   Fact: Many insurers cover the normal costs of treatment on cancer clinical trials, and many states have mandatory coverage.

standard of care for your type of cancer, it is more likely that you will be asked to participate in a Phase III or higher trial.

Phase I Trials don't mark the beginning of a drug's journey: To get to this phase, a treatment has already shown effective results on tumors in animals. In Phase I, researchers test a treatment on a small group of people to determine its side effects and safety and to learn of a safe dosage on humans. Patients in Phase I treatments generally haven't responded to customary therapies.

Phase II Trials extend the safety assessments of Phase I and further evaluate a treatment's effectiveness, including whether it might be successfully deployed against other cancers. Patient groups are larger than those in Phase I but still small, with a maximum of a few hundred.

Phase III Trials look for substantiation of the findings in the first two phases by comparing the treatment's results and side effects with that of the standard treatments. Groups are larger in Phase III, numbering up to three thousand.

Phase IV Trials nail down the final details of a treatment's best use in patients and more explicitly outline its risks and benefits.

6. **You need to be near a big hospital to take part in a clinical trial.**

   Fact: Many cancer clinical trials take place at local hospitals. Some also take place at local cancer clinics and doctors' offices.

7. **Clinical trials cost more than standard cancer treatment.**

   Fact: Not necessarily. Studies by groups including the American Association of Cancer Institutes, Kaiser Permanente, the Mayo Clinic, and Memorial Sloan-Kettering Cancer Center have found that the costs of routine care for patients in trials is comparable to the costs for patients not in trials. In addition, sometimes the hospital or drug manufacturer will compensate you for participating in a trial. Yeah, we know—it's still not worth having cancer.

8. **Once clinical trial participants sign a consent form, they must stay enrolled.**

   Fact: Not true. You can change your mind and not participate. You also have the right to leave a clinical trial at any time for any reason, without giving up access to other treatment.

9. **A clinical trial is a last resort in care.**

   Fact: Some people think that clinical trials are only a last resort after all other cancer treatments have failed. But they can often be a good way to begin treatment. As a cancer patient, you need to make sure you receive the best care from the very start.

10. **A patient needs the help of a doctor to begin to search for existing trials.**

    Fact: There are a number of free online search tools that allow patients to search for cancer clinical trials according to their type of cancer and ZIP code.

A gene therapy clinical trial must be approved by at least two review boards at the proposed institution, then be approved by the Food and Drug Administration, which regulates all gene therapy products.

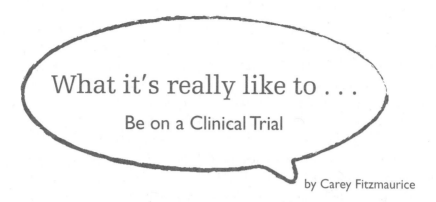

What it's really like to . . .

Be on a Clinical Trial

by Carey Fitzmaurice

My doctor told me that, unfortunately, the biopsy showed that my cancer had returned. It had been barely a year of remission.

But he had a plan. A great drug that was getting a lot of buzz. But it hadn't gotten FDA approval for my cancer yet (although it had been approved for others), so the only way to get it was a trial. There was one being done at my treatment center.

Now, my oncologist was telling me all this on the phone. He knew I wanted to know something ASAP. I had been carrying my phone around. I was in a meeting with some colleagues and a contractor. They knew I was waiting for this call.

Then started the waiting. To hear from the research nurse. Then the trial nurse. Then to go in and have all the tests run again. This was very different from my original treatment, which started right after my initial surgery. I knew that schedule right away, but for the trial I wouldn't know the treatment schedule until I was accepted and had started. Finally I was approved to start the trial, two months after I started the process.

I was warned that, since my insurance doesn't cover trials, there might be some expenses I'd have to pay. The doctor visits they would cover, as well as the CT scans that the protocol required. The drugs themselves would be covered by the trial. But the mixing of the chemo and the infusion I might have to pay for. About $1,200 per infusion. Either every two or every three weeks. OK . . . what's the point of retirement money if I am not going to live to retirement? I could use it for this. How long away was FDA approval?

I called everywhere I could think of to see if this denial of coverage was allowed—I mean, this is the treatment my doctor thought I should have! No dice.

As it turned out, being on the trial was great! I had a nurse to call/text with every little problem! I had lots of blood drawn the first few times, but I got to go to research phlebotomy and skip the lines! I got parking vouchers! *And* the drug worked, with very few side effects. *And* somehow (I haven't wanted to ask too many questions), the bills were paid!

Day to day, being on the trial was no different from "regular" treatment. My trial involved taking a drug orally, daily. I went in for an infusion of the second drug every other week. I went to the same infusion center where I had been treated before—with my same fave nurses! There were many people on the trial with my kind of cancer, since this was the only way for us to obtain the drug. A few of them I knew, either from support groups or for other reasons. We generally had the same treatment day, as they scheduled infusions for the oncologist's clinic day. So we were able to compare side effects, which of the medical staff we liked (there was a PA who rubbed us all the wrong way); we even carpooled.

All was well until one of the routine CT scans being done as part of the trial showed that I had developed a new primary cancer. So, I had to go off of the trial in order to have the surgery, which showed lymph node involvement. If I hadn't been on the trial, it would have been another couple of months until this other cancer was caught.

After that surgery I had regular old chemo again. Then six months with no evidence of disease. As I write, I have recently found out that another lymph node seems to be growing. This time my onc thinks that I am a good candidate for a different trial. This one is not at my treatment center. So I am now going through the major hassle of trying to get all my medical records, tumor blocks, radiology results, etc., over to the trial nurse. I have an appointment to go in and have an orientation on participating in the trial and to meet the clinical team. At some point they will let me know if I am approved.

Because everything having to do with research is regimented, in this trial they start new patients only on certain days (some trials start a new group every four weeks or every six). So, even if I get on the trial, I will have to wait for a slot on one of the start dates. My oncologist has said that there should be no problem for me medically to wait a couple of months to start. Then, it will be the same as starting chemo again, with infusions every three weeks and CT scans every six. But it will be worth it.

I hope that there are tissue samples left! I have authorized every study I've been asked to be a part of. If *anything* about my experience can be at all useful in finding better detection, better treatments, cures for either of my types of cancer, or the genetics involved so that others and their families don't have to go through any of this, please use it all. I have benefited from everyone who participated in trials that led to the approval of the standard drugs and methods that have been used on me. I have benefited from the trial I was on before. I will continue to seek out the drugs and therapies that my doctors think will work for me—even if the only way to get them is to go through the upfront hassles of getting on a trial.

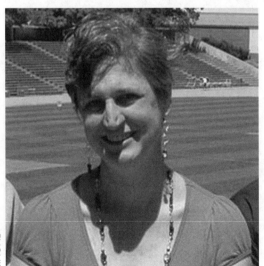

SIMONE

Guides
to the Planet

Diagnosed with Stage IIIC ovarian cancer at thirty-seven, Carey Fitzmaurice has had multiple recurrences; she has also been diagnosed with breast cancer. Carey is an active participant in the Ovarian Cancer National Alliance's Survivors Teaching Students program and is the founder of Teal Toes, an organization seeking to raise awareness of ovarian cancer.

{ The main ones fill up TV shows and movies, and they're for real: nausea, baldness, and fatigue. }

Chapter Four

Side Effects

During chemo I got so beaten down my friend got in touch with the hospital. They brought me in, gave me some fluids, and it wasn't long before I felt OK. I never would have called myself, and I was so far gone it could've been really, really bad had I not gone in. Bottom line is that you can combat side effects from chemo, sometimes pretty easily, especially if you involve your doctors and caregivers.

—MADMAX

Most of the time I'm too exhausted to even think about anything, as I'm expelling every possible liquid from my body. I need to vomit. I want to vomit. It makes the entire painful process complete. Instead, I just gag. I hang over the seat, sometimes groveling on the bathroom floor with my head on the toilet, praying that God will allow me to propel something from my body.

—ERIN SHMALO

The rock-solid foundation of chemo's formidable street cred is its side effects. The main ones fill up TV shows and movies, and they're for real: nausea, baldness, and fatigue. There are also lesser known but no less formidable frenemies—"frenemies" because, let's not forget, chemo is about ridding you of cancer, which is pretty cool—anemia, constipation, diarrhea, immunosuppression, chemo brain, and mucositis/stomatitis (mouth sores). Following is about as candid a discussion as you'll find about

chemo's side effects, including some tips from the Planet on how to deal with them.

Required caveat: The tips in this section aren't guaranteed panaceas (i.e., "cure-alls"; if you're reading this book, it's a word you should know); they're simply ideas that worked for at least one person on the Planet. To be sure, some items worked for many people—nonetheless, Planet Cancer cannot claim that the information here represents, supplants, outpaces, or wages war on medical data. Bottom line: As you adjust to living on the Planet, there's nothing that can take the place of your doctor. Except a hot date, a motorcycle trip along the Grand Canyon's rim, or perhaps another doctor of comparable competence. That said . . .

Nausea

Thanks to chemo, I'll never be able to enjoy butternut squash soup again. Same with Killian's beer, but that was due to a long game of quarters, not chemo.

—KATE THAXTON

Every time I use the restroom at the hospital and smell the hand soap, I almost puke. I have even thought about taking my own soap in my purse to avoid smelling it.

—LAB

Vomit, emesis, puke—whatever you want to call it, throwing up is the Mack Daddy side effect of chemotherapy. There are lots of tips for nausea suppression, but if you can't remember anything else, remember this: *Stay ahead of it.* There are lots of good drugs now for calming the retching seas in your belly, but a key factor is to take your meds before you're hanging over the toilet. Once nausea grabs hold, it can be awfully hard to get in front of it again.

One other very important rule about nausea and chemotherapy: Do not, under any circumstances, including the deepest cravings, eat your favorite foods during chemo! The taint they'll have after mingling with the chemicals will make you unable to eat them again, at least not for a long, long time.

How Nausea Is Treated on Planet Cancer

Don't get us started on the irony of antinausea meds that have to be taken by mouth, but suffice it to say that if you have difficulty getting a pill down and keeping it down, there is always the option of door number two. Suppositories are your friend, as are intravenous antinausea meds.

Antinausea drug candidates include the brand-name meds Zofran, Kytril, Ativan, Phenergan, and Emend, among others. Zofran also comes in a wafer form that you can dissolve under your tongue, and there's an antinausea patch called Sancuso that you can slap on your arm for five days of relief at a time.

There's also Marinol, an innocuously named pill that, though it conjures images of a senior citizens' community in Sarasota, is, in fact, a synthetic form of THC, the active ingredient in marijuana. There are those who swear that smoking the real stuff does wonders to soothe the anxiety, pain, and nausea wrought by chemo. The loudest proponents of smoking actual

marijuana cite its rare characteristic of boosting the appetite, which the antinausea drugs listed above make no official claim to do. (Some patients claim that Marinol boosts the appetite; others say no.)

Regardless, if you *are* partying with Mary Jane—for medicinal purposes or otherwise—be sure to tell your doctor, just as you would for any supplement, as it may interact badly with some antidepressants or other prescription meds. If you're gonna go after the real, smokable stuff, make sure you know the risks—marijuana smoke contains carcinogenic hydrocarbons, 50 to 70 percent more than cigarettes. This isn't

---

Tried-and-True Tips for Nausea

- Water can taste awful during chemo, and Gatorade packs on the calories. Instead, make iced tea with ginger tea—you can vary the strength to make it stronger or weaker. The ginger is an extra bonus (even if just a placebo) for nausea!

- I can't say enough about the Ginger People Ginger Chews for nausea.

- Nausea deterrents: dried mango, mint tea.

- Some cite acupuncture as having helped curb nausea.

- Carry a bag of lime/lemon rinds around with you and sniff it when you feel sick.

- Keep barf bags in the glove compartment of your car. You never know when the urge to (involuntarily) purge will strike.

A fine book by Dr. Dan Shapiro, *Mom's Marijuana*, discusses how his mom grew marijuana for him to help him control his nausea during treatment. We should all have moms like that.

good for you, despite the potentially beneficent nature of the smoke. You might get cancer from it! This is why many treating pain and nausea symptoms get around the carcinogenic down-side by using the marijuana in an edible form. Medical marijuana is legal in many states, and more have proposed legislation. Your doc will doubtless be familiar with the laws in your state.

Perhaps the most important thing to note here about antinausea medication is that there are many kinds. Some are listed above. One might not work well for you. If this happens, tell your doctor to try another. There's no reason to keep taking a med that doesn't work when others serve the same purpose.

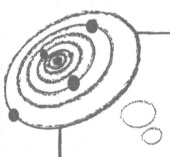

Dispatches from the Planet

I'll throw some things out there that worked for me:

- Not lying down. I try to prop myself up on the couch with some pillows, so I'm more sitting up than lying down, but still comfortable. That helps a lot. One of my first roommates in chemo told me this and it's always helped.

- Emend is such a lifesaver: It's a three-day pill you take during treatment. Honestly, it's the best. Also, when my nausea is raging, I have Ativan as a backup. There have been times when I've taken Zofran, Reglan, and Ativan each day—one every few hours, which keeps things at least manageable.

- Seltzer water (cold). Just plain seltzer with lemon, lime, mandarin, etc., flavor— whatever you like—but nothing with any aspartame or sweeteners. Something about it is pretty comforting. The bubbles settle my stomach, and the slight flavor of it helps—I have trouble drinking regular water since my mouth tastes like chemicals post-chemo, and it seems to cover it up and I can keep my fluid intake up.

- Tortilla chips. For whatever reason, a tortilla chip or two every half hour or so really seems to help things along. I think if I go too long without eating, my stomach starts to become more prone to waves of nausea. I find that, if I eat just a bite or two here and there, I can keep the nausea at bay. I have no idea why tortilla chips, but it's just been one of those random things I discovered along the way.

- Fresh air. When things are really bad, I head outside for a minute and get out of the stale indoor air. If nothing else, it takes your mind off the nausea.

Nausea is a bit of a head game, so even if things seem minuscule, perhaps just the act of trying to be proactive and taking steps to keep it under control will in itself be helpful.

—*Attica*

For some reason I never got sick after chemo if I ate really heavy, fatty comfort foods like mac-n-cheese, fettuccini carbonara, mashed potatoes, etc. Yes, my waistline suffered (all the steroids didn't help either), but it was the only thing that kept me from puking my guts out.

—*Shannon E. Ford*

I used constant self-acupressure to ward away my nausea and prevent puking. I worked the stomach meridian. (I don't have any big beliefs in chi or energy work—all I know is that this worked for me!) First I stroked my bottom ribs from the center out toward my sides, slowly and gently. Then I pressed down the shins

of each leg in a gentle motion from knee to ankle repeatedly in a rhythmic pattern (never upward from ankle to knee because you want to move the "energy" down and out). Then I massaged the second toe next to the big toe, the toenail and corners of the toenail are most important. Again always massaging outward to the end of the toe rather than back and forth.

—*Kairol Rosenthal*

Avoid hot baths. Dramatic temperature change can make nausea much worse.

—*Rachel*

Alternative Terms for Vomiting

- Be the Exorcist
- Blow Chunks
- Peristalic Pyrotechnics
- Hurls
- Spew
- Yack
- Snarf (involves nasal output)

The Secret of One Person Who Didn't Puke During Chemo

by Donzie

Having been one of the few, the proud, the pukeless, and not knowing whether it was the antinausea meds, genetics, my nutritionist's strategy, or all three that contributed to this phenomenon, it's my duty to share the only thing I can: my nutritionist's strategy for what to eat and drink on chemo day. If this helps one person not puke for ten minutes, I'll be happy. Being a small bunny myself, this plan probably doesn't include enough food for a lot of you. Just try out what bits and pieces you think may work. You'll need:

- Dr. Lee's Organic Green Tea (loose) and a small strainer or tea ball

- Ginger root

- Ginger candy or chews, such as Reed's Ginger Candy Chews

- A blender or juicer (optional)

- Carrots, celery, cucumbers, beets

- Organic vegetable and/or chicken soup

- Turmeric or paprika

Before Chemo:
- Have a nice big mug of the green tea.

- Chew on pieces of ginger root (I didn't eat anything else before chemo).

During Chemo:
- Bring some of the ginger candy to chew or suck on.

- Two sixteen-ounce bottles of water; slowly sip, just let that chemo do its work and pee it out as quickly as you can before it can hang out in your body and do unnecessary damage.

After Chemo:
- With the juicer, juice together some carrot and ginger for an after-chemo cocktail. Or carrot, ¼ beet, a cucumber, and celery. Or just buy premade juices—juicers can be difficult to clean, and who feels like cleaning after chemo?

- Enjoy the vegetable or chicken soup; include dark green veggies in the soup if possible. Season lightly with the turmeric or paprika.

- More water, water, water. Pee out that stuff. It's strong; it doesn't need to linger in your body.

My chemo was from 10 a.m to 1 p.m., so I used to have a light dinner in the evening. I hope this can help you on the road to being puke-free!

The Other End

The one thing that really stands out about my chemo treatments is that they always gave me some sort of drug before each one. They called it "hot pants," but I always thought that term was putting it much too mildly. For me, it felt like someone was putting out a cigar in my asshole! Although the feeling only lasted about fifteen seconds, it totally sucked and I couldn't dump right for about thirteen days—just in time for another treatment.

—Shannon E. Ford

News flash: Chemo also affects pooping—one day diarrhea, the next, constipation. Hey, what do you want? Cancer is, to invoke an erroneous stereotype, an older person's malady. Why not throw in an older person's plumbing? Diarrhea floods the system because your intestinal lining is constantly replenishing, and chemo drugs have a field day with cells that operate that way. As a Planet Cancer doctor sagely remarked, "Damage these cells and pass the Imodium."

As for constipation, your gut has many nervous system connections. Many narcotics as well as several chemotherapy drugs (such as vincristine for lymphoma or Taxotere for breast cancer) can affect the nerves. Chemo-induced constipation is a kind of temporary nerve damage to the gut. Several remedies are offered by veterans of the Planet below, but if all else fails there's always—white blood cell and platelet counts allowing—the ol' standby: the enema.

Yes, pooping is a funny topic, but it's definitely something to take seriously. Constipation and diarrhea can cause hemorrhoids and/or anal fissures, which are not funny at all. They can be difficult to treat when your immune system is on the fritz and can become chronic, lasting well beyond your treatment. A good (well, bad) example of a side effect's side effects! Stay on a good, regular (pun intended) bowel management program to avoid this pain in the ass (pun intended).

Even when nothing solid is being produced (or blocked), stay on the alert for chemo farts. Chemo kills indiscriminately—both your cancer cells and a lot more, including the bacteria in your intestines that regulate things when you're in a more normal state than, say, dealing with a bunch of toxic chemicals in your body. When your intestines' bacterial equilibrium is disrupted, you guessed it:

Helping Your Plumbing

1. Senna tea.

2. Prune juice unclogs intestines like magic, but it ain't the nectar of the gods: The secret to getting it down is to drink it really cold, over ice.

3. Magnesium tablets are good if you can't hack the taste of prunes.

Hot pants, or, alternatively (and no more medically), "ants in your pants," likely refers to Decadron, a widely used steroid that can have the cigar-in-asshole effect if pushed too quickly into an IV.

---

chemo farts. Not only are chemo farts notable for volume and frequency, but also for their otherworldly aromas. They are, after all, chemical creations.

Customarily, to sort out intestinal woes, your doc will deploy over-the-counter medications like Imodium, Senokot, Ex-Lax, Pepto-Bismol, etc.—you'll also be encouraged to drink lots of water, which is advice to be taken seriously, or with a few million grains of Metamucil. In more serious cases, they may resort to prescription medications, IV fluids, or an enema. So drink lots of water, don't forget the fiber, and keep a good magazine nearby.

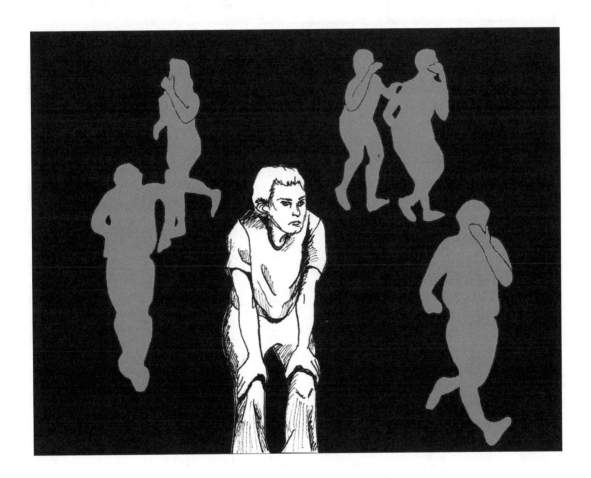

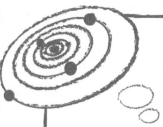

Dispatches from the Planet

After my third chemo I was regularly waking up my girlfriend in the middle of the night. I could sing and beat box with my ass. My beautiful, shiny, hairless ass. I lost shame about it. I never held 'em in. I'd waited a lifetime for this privilege.

—Fez

I am something of an expert on the subject of my own bowel movements. One of the more unexpected and bizarre transformations that my body underwent via chemotherapy was, sometimes, to produce frighteningly perfect bowel movements.

Through my three cycles of bleomycin, etoposide, and cisplatin chemotherapy, my bowels followed the same schedule. During the first week, I had partial constipation. With great effort, I would expel a handful of rounded little turds. During the third week, I would have fairly normal feces as my body began to recover from that cycle's dose of chemo. It was in the middle, during the second week, when things got interesting. I excreted a massive, unbroken horse dropping of alarmingly flawless composition and shape. The color, an odd hue of grayish-brown, was the only imperfect thing about it. Otherwise, it was suitable for framing. But it was also inhuman, without any of the flaws and foibles that give a normal turd personality and humanity; it looked like what a robot would shit if robots shat. Even now, it terrifies me to look back and contemplate the mixture of chemicals at work in my stomach that produced those bizarre uber-turds.

—Curtis Luciani

Miralax, aka Miracle-AX, is the best over-the-counter laxative out there. It is stimulant- and cramp-free, will not keep you up, can be dosed according to your needs, is flavorless, and can be mixed with any liquid or beverage.

—Rachel

Popular Culture's Finest Misrepresentations of Young Adult Cancer

We scoured all of pop culture to put together this list, which highlights some of the best (read: worst) depictions of young adults with cancer. It's doubtless incomplete, which says a lot about the popular conception of how cancer affects young adults.

Culprit: *Love Story*
Genre: Movie, 1970

- **Distilled Plot:** Rich boy (Ryan O'Neal) meets poor girl (Ali MacGraw). She can't get knocked up and, they learn, is dying of a terminal illness. (It goes unnamed but is understood to be leukemia.) Life lessons, not to mention the bizarre line "Love means never having to say you're sorry," ensue.

- **Misrepresentation of Cancer:** Ali Mac-Graw dies a quick, painless, peaceful death, and looks gorgeous as she hugs O'Neal and expires in the hospital.

- **More Realistically:** Come on—we've gotta explain this?! Also, love doesn't mean never having to say you're sorry; love means never having to shut the bathroom door.

Culprit: *Grey's Anatomy*
Genre: Television series, 2005 season

- **Distilled Plot:** An attractive, in-shape, and multiracial group of interns, residents, and doctors, including Meredith Grey, the title character, practice medicine and adulthood in a Seattle hospital. Complications set to alternative music ensue.

- **Misrepresentation of Cancer:** We're focusing exclusively on the show's misrepresentations of clinical trials. Here are a few, taken from different spots in various episodes:

Doctor: "No one cares about your clinical trial and your sick, sick, terminal patients, who would be better to be left for dead."

Doctor: "I am killing people for sport."

Patient: "Hey, brain butcher. . . . Cool, I'm your lab rat."

Doctor: "In a clinical trial, I am experimenting, groping around in the dark."

Doctor, referring to a clinical trial: "We kill things. We have killed twelve people and now we will kill a thirteenth."

Spoken words aside, also worth mentioning is the common montage of flatlines.

Culprit: *Degrassi High*
Genre: Television series, various years and iterations, beginning 1989

Distilled Plot: Issue-focused teen drama set in Toronto, Canada. Above-the-border scholastic dorkiness ensues.

Misrepresentation of Cancer: Degrassi has had a few efforts addressing cancer. In one, the school bully, Spinner, starts to fight after school while being videotaped. He gets Internet fame, he gets girls, he gets respect, and he gets sharp pains in the groin that prevent him from punching hard; his aggression increases after he gets diagnosed. He calms down after he has one of his testicles removed. And to fight back . . . he becomes a pothead. He also hangs out in immune system–compromising pubs at night while wearing a mullet/hat wig and complaining about his early morning chemo sessions before school. (Are you wondering why he's still in school, too?)

More Realistically: Picking fights and going to bars while in high school—could be realistic, but immediately post-seminoma, and without missing any class?

Culprit: *A Walk to Remember*
Genre: Movie, 2002

Distilled Plot: Popular aimless boy, forced to be in the school play, falls for quiet minister's daughter. Complications ensue.

Misrepresentation of Cancer: Mandy Moore, playing the preacher's daughter, has leukemia. She gets pale. That's it. She still has the energy to sing in the church choir, tutor delinquent youth, and star in the school play.

More Realistically: Place Moore on a couch in front of a television, wondering where the remote sitting on her lap has gone. She locates the remote when it falls to the floor after she jumps up to vomit. Optional: ear bleed, nose bleed, and two black eyes.

Hair Loss

It's weird. Early on I didn't want to be bald, not so much because I cared but because I thought it created awkward moments with other people, like they were uncomfortable; this, I learned, isn't even a little bit true. I ended up going bald most of the time. Nobody cared, including me.

—KRISTIN

I walked into a record store once on a hot Texas summer day without anything on my head. Totally bald, of course. The guy behind the counter said, "You look like Sinéad O'Connor." I said, "It must be the mouth."

—HL1994

After I lost my hair, I got a henna tattoo painted all over my head. It was awesome.

—CAREY

Even though chemotherapy doesn't cause hair loss in every instance, the bald person remains the unassailable symbol of cancer. It makes sense: Hair loss, or alopecia, is cancer treatment's most visible mark. Scars can come from any number of sources, and you can't very well pinpoint that someone who looks tired necessarily has cancer. But show us a twenty-five-year-old who looks as if he just had a full-body wax, including the nose hairs, and we'll show you somebody in the thick of chemo. (*Note:* Again, patients on chemo don't always lose all their hair.)

For this reason, even though it's not exactly painful to lose one's hair, it sometimes hits harder emotionally—there's lively discussion among patients and doctors and therapists, not to mention on the Planet Cancer Web site, about whether this emotional hit is a result of baldness being, like, *OK, I've really got friggin' cancer*, or whether it's actually tied to vanity, appearance, etc., or some of both. (See "Fashion" and "Wigs" in chapter 5.)

Let's drop some science: Hair follicles share with cancer cells a tendency to multiply rapidly, and so are equally as susceptible to being stunted by chemotherapy drugs (and radiation, though radiation's effects are localized). The good news is that these cells repair themselves post-chemotherapy; the cancer cells, we hope, do not.

Unlike with nausea or intestinal maladies, there's not much to do to combat baldness: Take your insurance company up on its fairly standard offer to provide you a wig, become expert at selecting hats based on comfort rather than style (after a while you'll find yourself with many found at the sweet spot where these two things converge), rock hard with scarves and bandannas, have some fun with henna tattoos on your scalp. Do whatever feels right, and remember that often more than one thing feels right.

{ A Head-Shaving Party on Planet Cancer }

by Jen Singer

When I started finding hairs in my Cheerios, I knew it was time. Just days after I'd finished my first round of chemo—a five-day infusion in the hospital—my hair started to fall out, little by little. I found it on my pillow. I found it on the shower floor. I found it inside my shirt. And then I found it in my Cheerios. So, I scheduled a head-shaving party.

I suppose most women would prefer to shave off their hair in private or to wait for it to fall out on its own, but I wanted to beat the chemo to it. I suppose it was my way of saying "Up yours" to cancer. Every time I absentmindedly ran my fingers through my hair, it came out in clumps. My scalp hurt like after a bad perm, and what was left of my hair had turned much darker than its usual dirty blond. I needed to feel a little bit in charge when everything was falling apart.

Friends and family gathered in my kitchen the Saturday before Fourth of July for the big Shave-

Off celebration. We had just cleaned out our cabinets to prep the house for remodeling in what must have been the greatest metaphor ever: The house and I were both under construction.

I sat in a chair, draped a beach towel over me, and handed my husband, Pete, the scissors. He seemed oddly giddy to do the honors, and frankly, I don't want to know why. First, he trimmed my hair while people took pictures. Then he shaved it until I had a swath of hair down the middle of my head. I grabbed my hair gel—I wouldn't need it again for another eight months—and spiked my hair up into a Mohawk "Mom!" I shouted. "I've quit school to join a punk band in London."

My mother smiled. "That's nice, dear."

If only I had thought of it when I was a teenager. I wondered, *Suburban moms don't wear Mohawks, do they?*

I took a deep breath and gave Pete the go-ahead. He finished shaving off the rest of my hair until I was bald, except for a five o'clock shadow. I looked in the mirror and quickly realized that I looked like an extra on *Star Trek: Voyager*. I should have kept the Mohawk, except I like my Cheerios without hair.

In a sign of solidarity, my friend and fellow soccer coach, Dmitri, had his head shaved, too. Now we looked like two extras from *Star Trek* or the "Before" picture in a Sy Sperling ad for couples.

That was it. I was bald. And I would stay bald for much of the rest of the year. Mostly, I hid it under a headscarf, though my kids didn't seem to mind when I went bald on hot summer nights. My hair finally started to grow back in November—the day after I went as Dr. Evil for Halloween. By March, I had a cute, very short hairdo, but it wasn't enough for a Mohawk. Not yet, anyway.

> **Heed the tips for ADD-type stuff, such as writing everything down (on a PDA or other such device), so that you always have access to it. Word games and sudoku will also help exercise your brain.**

FATIGUE

This feeling shouldn't share a word with what soldiers wear in combat. It needs its own word, like gravityhitsmelikeanuclearreactor. Sometimes I feel like I can't even lift my head. It's like you're so tired that it makes you tired.
—JOHNNYTHREESTEPS

You'll notice that references to fatigue appear frequently throughout this book. It's a side effect common to many treatments, and it is no joke. It's not "being tired." Cancer-related fatigue is to being tired what a starving lion is to your housecat. It will devour "being tired" and sleep on top of it for four days, with a side of space-out thrown in along with it if you're not careful.

Fatigue is an especially common symptom of anemia (see later in the chapter); it also sometimes shows up simply because your body is reacting to chemotherapy, like hey, I can't be 100 percent here if you're filling me with all these toxic chemicals which, by the way, might be putting some serious mileage on my heart and kidneys, so I'm going to dial it down for a month or two. This also explains how some patients experience fatigue long after treatment.

Fatigue is mercurial. You might feel pretty good one day, then get knocked sideways the next. One thing you can expect, though, is that your fatigue will actually become more consuming as your treatment continues. If you're aware of this, you can plan your days better, without being overambitious—you know, do a single, simple thing, like putting away your sweaters or meeting a friend for coffee, instead of a long list of errands that you'll be unlikely to complete (thus pissing yourself off).

So how to stave it off? Opinions vary, but the most consistently championed way to rip your fatigue out of that divot in the couch and slap its recalcitrant butt into gear is by exercising. Some people say that hormone medication helped them, some say certain vitamins, etc., but exercise reigns supreme. Check with your doc to develop a regimen that works for you to stave off fatigue, and see also "Exercise" in chapter 5.

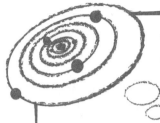

Dispatches from the Planet

It wasn't so bad at first.

In the beginning of my fourteen-month stint of chemotherapy, I'd be out of action for a few days after a treatment, then back on track. I was still working. Still spending time with my friends. Still running errands for my mom. As time went on, though, the "bouncing back" part seemed to get harder and harder. My blood counts took longer and longer to recover, and the intervals in between my treatments became longer and longer too.

It was a slow, cumulative snowball of fatigue. After every chemo session, I was able to do a little bit less. Every bout of fever, every transfusion— each one slowed me down just a little more. I had to stop working. And as the months went on, I had to make the call more and more often: "I'm sorry, I'm just not feeling up to dinner/a movie/a cup of coffee today." Gradually, I became more careful about even making a commitment in the first place.

I started to hoard my energy like a man lost in the desert does his water, rationing every drop, making no heedless withdrawals that would leave me empty. Every morning I would wake up and assess my energy levels and what I absolutely had to do that day. And by "absolutely had to do," I mean, "did I have a doctor's appointment." After that, I tried to do some sort of exercise, whether it was ten minutes on the treadmill or a walk around the apartment complex. If I still felt up for anything else, I'd get together with a friend for a brief, spontaneous visit.

Then again, there were days when I got up, looked in the mirror, and made the call: "It's just not gonna happen today." And it was back to bed to try and replenish the energy stores for the next day.

By the time I finished treatment, the question I asked myself every morning had become, "What is the ONE thing I want or need to do today?" The long months of treatment had taken a toll almost without my seeing it happen. But the light was shining at the end of the tunnel and I knew that I was almost there.

After I finished chemotherapy, I made the classic rookie mistake over and over of pushing it too hard, too fast. An afternoon out with a friend would lay me out for two days. I was so anxious to reenter the highway of my life that I ignored all the signals my body was giving me to rest, wait, recover. As my doctor pointed out, it took me many months to get to this point, and I should allow just as long to get back.

Slowly, slowly, I started feeling like myself again. After a few months, I could do more than one thing a day—after six months or so, I could do two, three, or even FOUR things a day! Victory! It took me more than a year before I could claim something close to normalcy again in terms of my energy levels, but I finally got there.

Now, years later, when people say to me, "I'm tired," I chuckle to myself sometimes. I think, "You know what? You have no idea."

—*hl1994*

Chemo Brain

I told someone that my birthday is March 31 the other day. It is actually March 30.

—LAB

Chemo brain is an aptly named phenomenon, one poorly understood but very real. To wit: "Where did I leave my keys?" "When the hell is the appointment?" "Are you my child?"

Everybody has these lapses, chemo or not, but chemotherapy can actually cause temporary cognitive dysfunction. Oncology is transitioning toward more targeted therapy (see "The Future: Gene Therapy, Targeted Therapy" in chapter 3), but most chemotherapy still involves toxic substances that affect both cancer cells and the normal body at different rates. Chemo brain, then, is the unwanted toxic effect of chemotherapy on brain function.

The largest studies about chemo brain have been performed in women undergoing adjuvant (postsurgical) chemotherapy for breast cancer. Cognitive problems may be subtle and are best detected with sophisticated neuropsychiatric tests. Patients explain the fuzziness with remarks such as:

"I just don't think as clearly."

"I'm not as sharp."

"Sometimes I think my foot is Andre the Giant."

"I forget things."

"Is this premature Alzheimer's?"

Take comfort: For the vast majority of patients, this fog does indeed dissipate after therapy is complete, though it can take up to a year to feel "normal." Exercise and a healthy diet appear to be helpful in restoring a chemo-addled brain, so don't think it'll all get better while you eat Cheez Doodles on the couch and watch *Scary Movie*. If you're already in the thick of it, let's say it again: Attention to nutrition and exercise can compensate for the effect of chemotherapy on cognition.

Research in another field, dementia in the elderly, has shown that those who "exercise" the mind by reading or doing brain stretchers such as crossword puzzles are less likely to experience decline.

Suggestions from the Mayo Clinic for Dealing with Chemo Brain

- Decrease workload.

- Avoid multiple tasks.

- Prepare today for tomorrow.

- Make lists.

- Sleep more.

- Use mnemonics and wordplay.

- Use (electronic) calendars to record appointments.

- Color-code and label items.

- Track memory problems in small diaries.

- Do crossword puzzles and sudoku squares to keep the mind sharp.

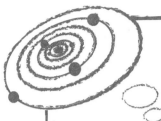

Dispatches from the Planet

After my AML [acute myelogenous leukemia] treatment in 1998, I wanted to go directly back into normal life. I was a great student before my treatment, but I found that I just could not function as I had before.

I thought I was just being spacey. My math facts would come and go in algebra, making my teachers wonder if I was adept to handle the work. I would also forget deadlines or do homework and forget to turn it in. My handwriting got really scratchy, and I had trouble understanding logical lessons in school. Not only did this last for two years, but also I literally felt like my brain forgot what school was.

Eventually, my teachers wanted to hold me back because they thought I wasn't as fast as the other kids. My oncologist and the hospital social worker stepped in and saved me from being labeled a student at risk. Although they didn't call it chemo brain at the time, they were the catalysts in proving to the school that the problems I was having were medical. My teachers became sensitive to my situation and adjusted their teaching styles, and I went to tutoring for further support.

I'm a senior in college now and I still at times feel the lingering effects of chemo brain, but I've realized the best thing to do is to talk about it and not stress about the way I'm functioning.

—*Cambrey Thomas*

I told my roommate, "It's like beating a dead . . . bush." I knew enough to ask for the right word, "horse." And then I said, "The aphasia as a side effect is really getting to me lately. Like can you believe I just got the 'Beating a dead dog' saying wrong?" And then they said, "Horse!"

I can effortlessly recall the word "aphasia"—a medical term referring to problems with language and memory retrieval and recognition—but common sayings are all jumbled.

—*Christy O'Connor*

I can't even cite just one incident because it happens all the time. The *worst* is when I was with a very good friend of mine after a radiation treatment, and I kept referring to my best friend's wife by the name of his ex-girlfriend. I guess I did this for about an hour, and no one had the guts to say I was using the wrong name. *Ugh!*

—*Denny Tu*

Top 10 Ways to Deal with Chemo Brain

10. Swear to everyone that you were a blond before you lost your hair.

9. Tell people that your brain "temporarily shuts down during chemo to prevent excessive loss of brain cells."

8. Spend the next twenty minutes trying to actually remember and articulate No. 9.

7. When your brain gives out and you stumble over a sentence, look the person directly in the eye and say, "Did you catch all that?"

6. Wait, what was I talking about?

5. Look at your oncologist and say, "Whoa! You're treating me for what?!?"

4. Proudly announce, "At least it doesn't affect my ability to drive!"

3. (For the girls) Tell everyone it gives you a chance to live in a man's shoes for a change. (For the guys) Hey, now you have a legitimate excuse to forget birthdays and anniversaries.

2. Wait, what was I talking about?

1. When all else fails, pretend you're having flashbacks from 'Nam—even if you weren't born until 1982.

A twenty-five-year-old Hodgkin's survivor provided the raw funny-power for this top 10. Thanks, Bobbi!

'ROID RAGE

Yes, 'roid rage is very real. Luckily, that was my low point and I never went after purse-snatchers or gangsters, but along the way there was road rage, doctor rage, Bush rage, lady at the DMV rage, guy who was ridiculously slow at the ATM rage.

—MIRA ELIAS

My oncologist, one of those rare birds who actually listened to what his nurse had to say, walks in and says, "I heard you had quite a buzz from the Decadron."
Me: "BEFORE OR AFTER I DUG OUT ALL THE YAUPON IN THE FRONT YARD?" I rest my case.

—JODY M. SCHOGER

Steroids are a mainstay on Planet Cancer. Natural and synthetic steroids are used in treatment regimens, primarily for lymphomas and some forms of breast cancer and leukemia; they're also employed to reduce swelling around tumors (this is usually done with brain tumors, as there's a finite amount of acreage inside your skull) and sometimes simply to provide pain relief. The side effects produced by steroids are their most famous calling card. The two primary culprits are an appetite increase and, yes, 'roid rage (others include acne, immunosuppression, and higher blood pressure and blood sugar). Legions on the Planet have expressed their beefs with gaining weight because of steroids, and others have stories of flying off the handle on their spouses for folding the laundry differently or screaming at their kid's kindergarten teacher for no apparent reason.

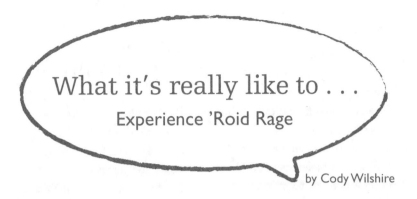

What it's really like to . . .

Experience 'Roid Rage

by Cody Wilshire

There are few things in life that can throw a survivor off his or her rocker. Once we get over that initial holy *bleep* moment, we tend to take everything else in stride, because, really, what other choice do we have? I was a trooper, I took it all with a grain of salt, I did my own research, I was as fully versed in all treatments as I probably could have been, when my doctor threw me for a loop: "We're going to put you on sixty mg of prednisone, daily, for at least two weeks."

OK, well, that can't be so bad, right? So it can change your emotions and give you nightmares. It can't be that bad, can it? Oh, it can. And it is. Prednisone has the magical power of turning the nicest person into someone who makes a hysterical pregnant woman look completely calm and sane. Thus with this wonderful drug that really does save lives comes what we lovingly call 'roid rage. How, you might ask? Well, for example, I love to cook. I really do. Who would have ever thought that being unable to sauté the onions just right could cause such a freak-out?

Let me rewind. My boyfriend loves to eat. I love to cook. Perfect relationship, right? Sure, if prednisone stays out of the mix. I was making spaghetti, a simple dish, with an old family recipe as the sauce. It's something I would make constantly, a fallback comfort food, and something I'm good at making. Chop, sauté, stir, boil, voilà—simple, right? Wrong. Add sixty mg of prednisone, very little sleep, and shaking hands to the simple task of chopping an onion and you will have one twenty-two-year-old woman screaming at the cutting board and yelling at her knife, begging it for an answer to the question: "Why are you doing this to me?! Why can't you just work like you always have done?! What did I ever do to you to deserve this?!" This all would be highly entertaining if I hadn't been dead serious.

My boyfriend came into the kitchen, excited I was making dinner, to find me leaning over the countertop, bawling my eyes out. He rushed over, like any good supportive boyfriend would do, and wrapped me up in his arms, asking me what was wrong. I couldn't really get anything out between the sobs besides "onions" and "The knife hates me. It wouldn't let me chop!" He let out a giggle, which, of course, made the tiny episode quickly turn into something quite large. "How is this funny to you?! Don't you understand how devastating this is to me? This is what I can do, this is what I'm good at, and I can't even freaking *chop* anymore! *Everyone hates me!*"

Poor guy. There was arm flailing and more tears, followed by me dramatically grabbing all the poorly chopped onions and throwing them in the pan to sauté, tossing my body against the countertop, and screaming dramatically, "I don't even care anymore! Just take them all away!"

Again, this all would have been quite entertaining if I wasn't dead serious. Needless to say, like the good boyfriend he was, he threw it away . . . and ordered a pizza.

Guides to the Planet

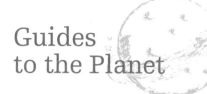

Cody Wilshire, known as "Dee," writes: "Dee. twenty-three. I am a survivor of multiple diseases. First diagnosed at age eighteen. Last diagnosed yesterday. I have a very strong grasp of who I am; it will never waver. I am a strong-minded, steadfast individualist. Proud eco-ist, foodie, music snob, and animal lover. Anything I set my mind to, I will do. That is all."

Immunosuppression

Your immune system is compromised to varying degrees during chemotherapy, largely for the same reason we've discussed regarding hair loss, nausea, and intestinal problems: The cells that compose your immune system are rapid dividers, and these types of cells get hit hardest by the toxic chemicals patrolling your insides.

Chemo retards the functioning of your bone marrow, the engine that runs your immune system. When you receive chemo, your red blood cell counts become lower (result: exhaustion and anemia); your white blood cell counts become lower (infection and illness); and your platelet counts become lower (trouble with blood clotting).

Odds are high that during some point of your treatment, your white blood cell count will plummet and you will be deemed "neutropenic." Roughly translated, this means that your immune system is now a six-year-old pipsqueak getting trampled on the swarming, no-holds-barred varsity field of infection.

The general rule to keep in mind: Keep everything around you—including people—disinfected, and watch what you eat, touch, and swallow. Avoid salad bars and buffets. Switch seats in the movie theater if someone is coughing behind you—or, better yet, sign up for Netflix or get a DVR and stay home. Buy stock in companies that manufacture Purell and Lysol, because you will be singlehandedly boosting sales. (*Note:* If you use Lysol or other products to clean, rinse off your food-preparation areas to ensure that the chemicals stay clear of your dinner.) Get a T-shirt that reads, "I'm neutropenic, and if you can read this, you're *too close!*"

Just kidding. But seriously, there's no shame in being the boy or girl in the bubble for a while. Better safe than infected.

A Helpful Checklist for Self-Injection

If your immune system goes down for the count at any point, you'll doubtless have to give yourself some shots. The shots are typically of G-CSF (shorthand for granulocyte colony stimulating factor; brand name Neupogen or Neulasta), drugs that boost your immune system.

> Keep everything around you—
> including people—disinfected,
> and watch what you
> eat, touch, and swallow.

When you're *neutropenic,* your doctors may put you on a special diet for suppressed immune systems. The neutropenic diet is rich in well-done meats, overcooked eggs, and canned fruit, and contains no fresh fruit and vegetables. The bacteria-free neutropenic diet is standard both before and for a few months after transplants. (Of note: the overwhelming lack of neutropenic diet–themed restaurants.)

Self-injection is tough for a lot of reasons: It's not a particularly natural thing, this poking needles into yourself, and many are squeamish about it. Especially at first, it's something you're scared of messing up (e.g., "What if I inject this stuff somewhere that hurts me?"). It's precise, a little tedious, and just not one of the more fun aspects of cancer treatment.

With these and the other touchy factors in mind, we asked Greg Ferris, transplant veteran, to give us a primer on what you should know about self-injection. Below is all the wisdom you could possibly want about self-injecting. Thanks, Greg.

One more thing: Make sure you're trained by a member of your health-care team, and don't do it yourself until you are comfortable with the process. Greg's words, though sage, should not be used as a replacement for appropriate training from your health-care professional.

{ Self-Injection and How to Do It }

by Greg Ferris

The first step in the injection process is to find out where you stand psychologically. Many people fear needles. (Don't assume you don't until you've had to inject yourself.) If you do, don't feel guilty about asking for help. Most shots can either be given at your clinic or by a friend/spouse/caregiver who has been appropriately trained. After all, nothing says "I love you" more than "Hey, honey, can you come stick me in the ass?"

Isolate a place in your home as your injection area. Choose a place like a desk or table in a guest room that is not associated with pleasurable activities. To avoid falls, make sure you have a sturdy seat.

Before you start, make sure you are physically stable enough to be giving yourself an injection: Your platelet count is high enough; you are not having episodes of dizziness, fainting, lightheadedness, etc. If you live with others, make sure they know you are about to give yourself your shot, and not to interrupt.

Make a checklist of all the necessary supplies you need to have: a needle, a syringe, alcohol wipes, medication, a sharps disposal container. You don't want to be halfway through the process and realize you are missing something. Review the checklist before beginning each injection until it becomes second nature to you.

Wash your hands thoroughly before beginning and have antibacterial gel handy so you can continue to sanitize if needed throughout the process. If you wear contacts or glasses, make sure they are at hand.

Clean the desk or tabletop thoroughly. A good wipe-down with a Clorox wipe will suffice, but don't forget to also wipe the chair arms, the lamp you might be using, etc., as they all could be potential contaminants. After wiping down the area, I have always taken the additional step of laying clean paper towels down on the surface.

Wipe the injection site with an alcohol wipe as well. The most common areas to self-inject are the upper thighs, the belly, and the butt. Depending on the frequency and type of injection, you will want to rotate injection sites and areas—some areas may bruise more easily than others. As a general rule, the "softer" the area (i.e., fatter), the less painful the injection. It sounds counterintuitive, but I have found that the stomach is least painful. It's a good idea to have full visibility—stomach and top of your thighs are best for that. If someone else is injecting you, the back of your arm (between shoulder and triceps), is also a good spot.

Prior to uncapping the needle, wipe the top of the medication vial with a fresh alcohol wipe. Do this before *every* insertion of a needle into the vial. You can leave an open alcohol wipe on top of the

vial(s) so that you are ready to wipe immediately before uncapping the needle.

If you are using pre-prepared syringes, take the top off the needle, pull back a bit on the plunger while pointing the needle skyward, then tap the syringe to work out any air bubbles. Slowly depress the plunger until there is no air left in the syringe, only medication. Check to verify that the dosage is correct.

For injections that require you to draw medication from a vial, attach the needle and then carefully pull the protective cap off. Once the cap is off the needle, pull back on the plunger, filling the barrel of the syringe with air equivalent to the dosage you need to draw from the vial (i.e., if you need 2 cc's of medication, pull back the syringe to the 2 cc level).

Hold the vial firmly on a clean, flat surface with one hand and insert the needle into the rubber top of the vial, being careful not to contaminate the needle by touching anything along the way.

Once the needle is in the vial, grab the vial with one hand, the syringe with the other, and turn the vial upside down. Push the predrawn air into the vial and then pull the plunger back to extract a bit more than the desired dosage. With the needle still in the vial, tap the syringe with your finger to drive air bubbles up to the top. Push the air bubbles and extra med back into the vial. (You can also remove the needle and push the air bubbles and extra meds out onto the paper towels, but don't touch the needle to the towels.)

Now it's injection time!

Some people find that pinching the area prior to giving the shot and/or taking a few deep breaths before the injection, then breathing out slowly during the injection, are helpful in reducing stress and pain. A smooth, quick motion is best—you don't want to prolong the discomfort by inserting the needle slowly (unless your doctor has directed you to do so), nor do you want to stab yourself.

As you're pushing the medication in, if you feel resistance, slow down. The thicker the medication, the slower you will want to push it in. Make sure you have given yourself the full dose required before removing the needle. Sometimes it is helpful to apply a little pressure or to rub the area a bit after injecting to help disperse the medication.

If you make a mistake and contaminate the needle, don't fret. Not a big deal. Just discard (see below) and start again. Do not reuse a needle!

If you have a specific sharps disposal container, discard the entire syringe immediately. Otherwise, be sure to re-cap needles before discarding them to avoid injecting your garbageman or a hapless homeless person. Don't try to put the cap back on freehand. Lay the protective cap down flat on your table/desk, then slowly slide the exposed needle back into the top. Only when the needle is safely back in the protective covering should you push the cap all the way on.

To review:

- Make sure everything is cleaner than you think it needs to be.

- Go slow and easy.

- Don't hesitate to ask for help if you need it. Some days you may want help more than others.

- Most important, don't worry about it. This is a long, detailed explanation of something that may take you all of two minutes on a good day.

Guides to the Planet

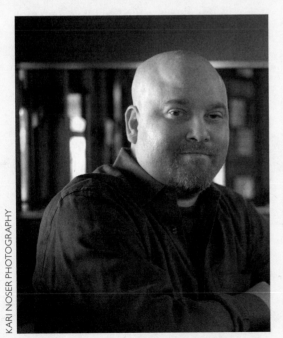

KARI NOSER PHOTOGRAPHY

Greg Ferris is the president and CEO of SWD Productions, LLC, an award-winning Houston-based independent film and video production company. Greg was happily leading a successful professional career in the structured finance business until his life path changed when he was diagnosed with leukemia in December 1999. After undergoing a bone marrow transplant in May 2000, he has spent nearly the last decade fighting for his life and fighting for the advancement of cancer research and quality-of-life issues for cancer survivors. He is also widely praised as the inventor of the Hairless Huddle, a key element of Planet Cancer's weekend retreats.

Self-Injection Tips

1. Request the thinnest gauge needle possible. The thinner the needle, the easier it is to insert and the less accompanying pain (many injections can indeed be close to pain-free).

2. Schedule your shot five minutes before your favorite TV show starts to force you to get it over with quickly.

3. Leave vials or prefilled syringes out of the refrigerator for five minutes or so, but not too long, to warm up before injecting and reduce the burning sensation.

4. Don't freak out if you get a giant bruise from a teeny-tiny shot. Thank your low platelet count.

Anemia

Red blood cells are single-purpose couriers in your body, delivering only one thing: oxygen. When you're going through chemotherapy, postal holidays go through the roof, red blood cells go on unacceptably long vacations, and oxygen doesn't get distributed throughout your body to any acceptable degree. When this happens, you likely have anemia.

Symptoms are feeling weak and/or cold and experiencing dizziness, pallor (pale skin), and fatigue. One way to combat anemia while you're undergoing chemotherapy is via blood transfusions, which replenish the red blood cells you need to adequately distribute oxygen throughout your body. Many doctors nowadays are more proactive, prescribing their patients drugs such as erythropoietin to jump-start red blood cell production and treat anemia.

Mucositis/Stomatitis: Mouth Sores

If you want to avoid mouth sores, begin by trying to brush your teeth. If you can't, get some antiseptic mouthwashes that don't have salt in them from a nurse. If throat sores come your way, you can't swallow pills or food.

—SEAN

Guess where else in your body is a source of rapidly dividing cells that can sustain collateral damage during chemotherapy? The gastrointestinal tract—specifically the mouth, throat, and esophagus. When doctors talk about "mucositis" or "stomatitis," they mean mouth sores. (Technically, stomatitis refers to sores in the mouth and mucositis refers to sores that occur in any mucous area, but try splitting that hair with a patient who has either.)

These sores, made up of inflamed tissue in the mucous membranes, are a fairly common side effect of chemotherapy and radiation to the gastrointestinal tract. Sometimes the sores can extend down into the throat, which is when you might hear the term "esophagitis." Besides swelling, symptoms can include dry mouth, chapped lips, and an altered capacity for tasting.

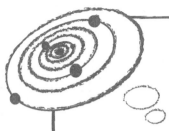

Dispatches from the Planet

Get lots of Clorox or Lysol wipes and use them often. It's really important to use them in the kitchen, eating areas, and the bathroom. If possible, have family members use a separate bathroom. Also, put bottles of hand sanitizer all over your house and have your family and visitors use them.

Keep your children away from sick people and sick people away from the house. Don't be shy about asking potential visitors forcefully about this, because I found that some of my friends were hiding illness symptoms because they really wanted to see me and didn't want to be turned away. I appreciated the thought, but really! I also required any visitors during the winter to have been immunized against the flu. I had my own couch in the family room that no one else used, so when my brother was coughing his lungs up, he wasn't getting it on my hangout area. Get Lysol or another spray that kills germs and spray chairs and couches after potential infections.

Then there is food preparation safety. Don't use your hands! Use tongs or food safety gloves. If it's absolutely necessary to use hands—like putting away slices of bread—have your spouse do it.

—*Mira Elias*

Regardless, *all* of these symptoms fall under the category of "suck-itis."

The downside of these mouth and throat sores—basic discomfort notwithstanding—is that they can affect your ability to eat and drink, and if you can't take in fluids and nutrients, your poor, beleaguered immune system will be worse off and you'll be more susceptible to infections.

There are nearly as many medical approaches to taking on mouth sores as there are hospitals. Oral medicines range from chlorhexidine, an oral antibacterial rinse, to nystatin, an antifungal medicine that can be taken in liquid or lozenge form, to other medicated mouthwashes that relieve pain, such as lidocaine elixir, morphine elixir, and a straight-up old-school saline swish. If pain is intense, some big guns—morphine or Dilaudid—might enter the picture.

Some tips from the Planet to prevent mouth sores from occurring or, if you have them, to keep from aggravating the pain:

- To prevent mouth sores from chemo drugs—this is prevention, not treatment—**suck red popsicles** (they have to be red!) beginning about fifteen minutes before the infusion,

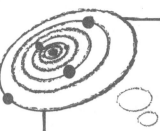

Dispatches from the Planet

I didn't know that I was anemic. I just knew that I was spending an inordinate amount of time lying on the bed watching shadows move across the walls while idly contemplating how long I could lie there until I absolutely had to get up to pee.

When I did get up, the lightheadedness always kicked in, hard. I had to grab something to steady myself while the blackness rolled away from my eyes. The dull headache remained, though, and the being cold. I could have filled Lake Erie with the amount of hot water I used up in shower time that year, trying to raise my core temp. And the fuzziness—oh, lord, the fuzziness. I couldn't concentrate at all. Read a book? Forget about it. I could barely make it through a fashion or gossip magazine, and that was just flipping through, looking at pictures.

When I finally went in for a complete blood count that first time around, they punted me over to the infusion room for the first of many transfusions that would take place over the course of the next year (back in the bad old days, pre-Epogen). I remember that I had on a hooded sweatshirt with the hood pulled up tight around my head to stay warm, so I was just peeking out of a small hole in front. I lay back in the infusion chair as they hung the bag of bright red blood, drifting in and out of awareness.

Gradually, though, as the blood dripped in, I started "waking up." I loosened the strings on my hood, sat up, and looked around. I stretched. I felt sharp. Smart. Energetic. The bag finished and they unhooked me. I high-fived the nurse, thanked her for clearly giving me the blood of some NBA all-star, and ran out of the hospital. It never felt quite that good again.

—*hl1994*

continually throughout it, and for about a half hour after it. The ice seems to constrict blood vessels and prevent irritation. The popsicle has to be red because other flavors of popsicles, such as lemon or lime, are too acidic.

- Along the same lines, **avoid citrus and acidic foods** (tomatoes, lemons, etc.).

- **Avoid spicy foods.**

- **Concentrated, cool chamomile tea** has a calming effect on ravaged oral tissues.

- **Brush teeth quickly** after eating (using a soft toothbrush).

- **Add half a teaspoon of salt, half a teaspoon of baking soda, and a splash of hydrogen peroxide to eight ounces of warm water.** Swish around in your mouth religiously after meals and before bedtime.

- **Avoid alcoholic and carbonated beverages as much as possible.**

Chemo-Induced Menopause and Vaginal Atrophy (Note: Not Two Punk Bands)

I tried to get it on last night and it killed.
Is this what they call vaginal atrophy?

—ALLISON

Chemo-induced menopause, or ovarian failure: How much fun can a cancer patient have? As follicles mature to release eggs, the cells in the ovaries constantly divide, so they are exceptionally vulnerable to chemotherapy.

The good news: You're finished with those mind-numbing monthly decisions of birth control, wings vs. no wings, thick and long (loofah pants) vs. oops, not thick and long enough.

The bad news: Your body slammed overnight into that estrogen-free era that most women take four years to gradually transition into.

The symptoms vary for every woman, but basically think Bikram yoga (the sweatbox variety) predicated by a nausea appetizer up to fifteen times a day—commonly called "hot flashes." These hot flashes, of course, can lead to irritability and make for some nice wig-throwing demonstrations in public places. Mood swings? Let's put it this way: If you were in the carnival, you could charge serious money for this ride. Oh, and it can last up to four years.

Some types of chemotherapy are more apt to induce menopause. For example, MOPP chemotherapy, an older treatment for Hodgkin's lymphoma, caused chemo-induced menopause in more than 90 percent of all young women.

ABVD, a newer therapy, preserves ovarian function in 90 percent of female patients.

In general, the closer a woman is to natural menopause or the more chemo regimens she has undergone, the greater chance that the process will be accelerated. Ask your oncologist about the specific chemotherapy proposed and about the known rates of chemo-induced menopause. Address symptoms of early menopause with your doc to ensure vaginal health and integrity.

Discuss whether hormone replacement is an option. If hormone replacement is not an option and hot flashes are interfering with your sex life, discuss medication and alternative options. Also, keep it in perspective (you ain't dead) and always have your glasses nearby—wine, that is.

Vaginal atrophy, aside from being a popular name for all-female a capella groups, is another side effect of chemotherapy that leads to painful sex. The ovaries fall prey to chemo's tendency to destroy all rapidly dividing cells. The ovaries produce estrogen, which is responsible for normal vaginal moisture, which, in addition to enabling good comfortable sex by stepping up lubrication naturally, protects against urinary tract infections. Vaginal dryness and pain with intercourse or urination are common side effects of declining estrogen levels during chemotherapy.

How to cope? Try a vaginal estrogen cream. These creams deliver a local estrogen effect to the vaginal mucosa—not your whole system. If you have breast cancer, discuss using this cream with your oncologist, as some breast cancers respond to estrogen. An approach that does not involve estrogen is to use a personal lubricant.

In many women, estrogen levels rise after the completion of therapy. In others, low estrogen persists. In essence, a young woman is experiencing what older women encounter after menopause. The fact that most postmenopausal women enjoy fulfilling sex lives proves the point that there is hope even if the transition is difficult.

Skin

Chemo cured my eczema.

—**LAB**

We know. You already graduated from teenage Clearasil days. Well, welcome back. On Planet Cancer, the odds are good that you'll have some whacked-out side effects from chemo and/or radiation that are going to play out a little cellular drama on your skin.

Because chemo also affects normal cells that grow quickly, such as skin cells, you should plan on suffering through at least one option or two off the delectable menu of itching, rashes, acne, sun sensitivity, and allergic reactions. If your chemo drugs leak from the cannula, your skin will burn and swell (doctor time!). Also, if you don't have a central line and the chemo is going in through a vein, the veins you use for treatment may darken up, but that'll fade within a few months post-treatment.

Some drugs, such as Adriamycin, can (temporarily) change the very hue of your skin. Many people report a reddish tinge, like being sunburned, to their face and/or hands after receiv-

> **A cannula** is not a creamy, sweet Italian dessert. It is, in fact, a tube that carries something into (or out of) your body.

> **Isotretinoin** (known also as Accutane) is a chemotherapeutic agent that has been used to treat severe acne for decades.

ing the drug, known also as "The Red Devil." Some people forego wearing contacts when being treated with Adriamycin due to the possibility that the lenses will be stained pink. (Seriously.) There have also been reports of red pee, pink and red sweat, and a persistent aversion to drinking any red liquids.

The good news about Acne, Part Deux, at this time in your life? Usually, all of these skin maladies are pretty manageable and fade about eight weeks after treatment. In the meantime, gentle, natural products will help keep things on an even keel. Use antibacterial soap and water-based moisturizer to help prevent infections and dry skin. Wear sunscreen and protective clothing, and don't forget the hat if you have virgin skin up there that's used to being covered by hair. Drink as much water as you can, and avoid hot baths (no matter how good they feel in the moment. Willpower!).

If you find yourself on the radiation bus instead of chemotherapy, your skin problems should be limited to the area being treated. Watch out for "radiation recall," which is when a previously treated site becomes irritated when chemo is later administered. Primary deterrent for radiation-related skin problems: depending on the radiation site, long sleeves or pants, socks, a hat—whatever it takes to cover it up. Sunscreen no matter what. And don't forget frequent moisturizing with gentle products to keep that tender skin as supple as you can.

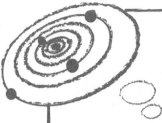

Dispatches from the Planet

My one bit of advice is something called Aquaphor. My radiologist recommended it to me, and it was wonderful in keeping my skin bearable. I would use it after every treatment, and I believe it helped from getting many burns.

—Gjaly

I swear it's true: Chemo cured my acne. Before chemo, I had to use Proactiv every day or my face would break out. Up until September, I had nice-sized blackheads that kept facialists busy. But now? Nothing. I don't need Proactiv, and my skin is blackhead-free and smooth.

—mommasaid

I just finished my eighth and final treatment of Rituxan for fNHL [follicular non-Hodgkin's lymphoma]. After the seventh treatment I got a rash over most of my upper body. It has not yet gone away, and since my treatment this week it has spread to the lower part of my body as well. I have talked with my nurse several times this week and she keeps telling me that the doctor says this is not uncommon and to take Benadryl until it runs its course.

—Barb Morse

My itchy, flaky psoriasis vanished during chemotherapy. And promptly returned along with my hair, but . . . I was OK with that.

—hl1994

Other Chemo Side Effects (in Case There Weren't Enough Already)

- **Bloating:** During chemo, you'll be hydrated with liters of saline. Some is peed out, and some your body absorbs—usually in your face, hands, and feet. This can lead to bloating. If your doctor determines that you're retaining too much fluid and you need help getting rid of it, you'll likely get a diuretic such as Lasix.

- **Blurry vision:** A temporary phenomenon described by some patients immediately after chemo sessions.

- **Hearing impairment:** Primarily associated with platinum-based chemotherapy drugs.

- **Neuropathy:** A problem of peripheral nerve function (nerves outside of the brain and spinal cord) that can result in a burning sensation, numbness, a "pins and needles" tingling, swelling, or muscle weakness.

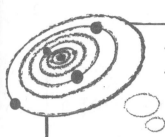

Dispatches from the Planet

During the later stages of my treatment, I started having serious issues with my bladder. It was terrible . . . sneeze and it was time to fetch a mop. I couldn't be more than ten minutes away from a bathroom because that is about how often I had to go. Most of the time it was just a trickle, but if I didn't want it down my leg, I needed to be close by at all times.

I was getting really freaked out. I was just sure that the radiation was frying my bladder and that I was going to have to wear adult diapers for the rest of my life. Then I found out that the antinausea medication Zofran has a side effect (if you take it for more than forty-five days) of *incontinence!* Man, as soon as I found that out I stopped taking it as quickly as I could. I was just about done with my part of the treatment that was causing nausea anyway. Within forty-eight hours the worst of my bladder problems was gone. I still don't have much of a warning, though, but it's getting better and better. (I can now go out in public!)

—*Talla*

What it's really like to . . .
Grow Moobies, or Man Boobs

by Justin Sullivan

So it appears I am turning into a woman! I was afraid of this when I found out that my sister was a match for the stem cell transplant.

I have been on this immunosuppressant, cyclosporine, that has a gang of terrible side effects.

1. I cannot be in the sun. If I do go outside for any period of time, I have to cover myself in sunscreen or wear long sleeves and a hat.

2. It speeds up the process of hair growth. This is not all bad, though, because all of my hair has grown back. However, I am now growing hair where hair did not grow before. And it is much thicker in all the other places. But this is something that we have experienced before. Hair never grows back the same after chemo. Now I just have to get my ears waxed!

3. This medication makes me vulnerable to infection, so even though I am getting healthier I still have to be very careful around people.

4. I am growing boobies!

Yes, boobies. If there is a one-in-a-million chance that it can happen, then it will happen to me. For good or bad. This time is no exception. There was a study done with this medication, and two men out of a shit ton of people grew breasts. They failed to mention this when they gave it to me due to the fact that it is so very rare. And now, I have titties!

At first it made my nipples very purple and sensitive. I complained about it a couple of times, and they said it would go away. A month later and . . . boobies. They are very small boobies, but boobies all the same. (Can you tell I like the word *boobies?*)

This "condition" is called gynecomastia (male breast enlargement). Fucking crazy. Funny as shit but not cool at all. When I was thirteen, I wanted breasts. But now that I have them, it's not as fun as I thought it would be. Fortunately for me I was able to convince the doctors that I wasn't making shit up, and they took me off the medication before you could even tell I had tits. They put me on some other medication. But the new medication is making me feel sick, so who knows. The irony of it all is that the first thing the doctor in Houston told me when we found out that my sister was a match was, "You will be a woman! Not on the outside. Just on the inside." It was funny when he said it, but now I am a little scared it might be true. Shit, what happens if I grow some ovaries or something?

{ Cyberchondria }

by Heidi Schultz Adams

One of the little known long-term side effects of cancer that we have discovered through purely anecdotal evidence on Planet Cancer is "cyberchondria." It's a tendency to self-diagnose with a multitude of illnesses, based on obsessive Internet research following symptom onset.

Cyberchondriacs are given to saying things like this: "Of course, the doctors don't understand. But *one day they'll see.* They'll see that *I was right all along!*" After all, you knew something was wrong the first time, right? No one believed you, but then it was cancer. So, in a way, cyberchondria is a protective mechanism to keep us from getting blindsided by that truck again.

I have a choice group of cyberchondriac gal pals. Can I just say how much I love these women!? For my last birthday, they gave me *The Complete*

Manual of Things That Might Kill You. How well they know me.

We validate each other's fears and support every attempt to get that test/scan/lab work, because . . . well, it's just therapeutic to take things to the worst possible scenario and then realize that your flesh-eating bacteria was just an infected pimple. An exercise in perspective, you might say.

A sampling of one of our e-mail conversations:

Liz: I've been having headaches, which is quite unusual for me; imagine my delight in connecting my recent trip to England to the eyeball-exploding pain. I had one bite of a very rare steak. Of course, Creutzfeld-Jakob disease, aka Mad Cow. Early symptoms? Insomnia, memory loss, depression, anxiety, withdrawal, fearfulness, and . . . headache. I'm done.

Stacia: Liz, sorry to hear about mad cow disease invading your body. Please be in touch before the hysteria takes over.

Jenny: I was bitten by fire ants Saturday afternoon and ended up in an ambulance. Thankfully I didn't die from the anaphylactic shock, or the panic. A pure shot of adrenaline seems to help with both of those conditions. In case any of you hypochondriacs ever need it, I now carry some in my purse.

Liz, maybe it can stave off the Mad Cow for a while; come on over and we'll give it a try.

Liz: So, you have an Epi-pen now? I got one after I had a systemic reaction to a penicillin-class antibiotic last year that was prescribed for the flesh-eating bacteria infection on my face.

Ahhhh, the power of shared imagination. Bring it on, folks—join the cyberchondriacs! We're waiting to hear from you and, yes, to tell you that we believe you, even if no one else does.

It's just therapeutic to take things to the worst possible scenario and then realize that your flesh-eating bacteria was just an infected pimple. An exercise in perspective.

Do not, under any circumstances, including the deepest cravings, eat your favorite foods during chemo!

{ The point is that, if nothing else,
having cancer illuminates
brightly the preciousness of
time, and you want to fill
this time up with stuff you like. }

Chapter Five

Staying Sane

Little by little, you will start to get pissed about being pissed, and you will be down. Let that happen, and turn this into what you never thought you could. You never expected to get crushed with all this, and the outcome of it will prove to be unexpected as well. But keep your head up, and get busy. Even if that means just walking around the block.

—LEFTY

As you navigate Planet Cancer, you cannot lose your hobbies—your penchant for mixing plaid shirts and pants, your need to sing and dance, your joy in bargain-hunting at the local mall, your workouts at the gym. What you're going through in treatment is serious stuff, sure. It's life and death. It takes all your energy and concentration, even as you feel both of those things taking unfairly long sabbaticals from your body and mind. But come on. What fun is the life you're struggling to save if you don't enjoy it even as you fight?

If you're a writer, keep a journal or contribute a hospital column to your local paper. Buy some big canvases and paint away if that's your bag. If you're a climber, find a manageable path up a mountain—and don't sweat whether or not you get to the summit! Photographers, document your treatment, or everything that isn't. Do yoga. Chat with the mailman. And don't forget to laugh whenever and wherever possible.

We on the Planet firmly believe in acknowledging both the ups and the downs—the fear and anger is just as much a part of this as the joy and laughter. It's called the human experience. But while we are most definitely not members of the scarily chipper "Positive Attitude Brigade," there is something to be said for filling your time with positive things, people, and experiences that you take pleasure in. You'll probably notice that it helps in dealing with treatment and post-treatment.

Keeping happy is a personal thing, obviously. What makes you happy? Only you know, and you should spend some solid time considering this important item during and after your treatment. We're not talking about "ending world hunger" or "climbing Mount Everest"; these things can be more along the lines of "being outside" or "perusing *TV Guide*." The point is that, if nothing else, having cancer illuminates brightly the preciousness of time, and you want to fill this time up with stuff you like.

What you'll find as you persist in your hobbies, in things that engage your mind and your spirit, is that the very things you think you don't have the energy to keep doing will have a big role in helping you heal.

Below are some suggestions based on what's worked for other people. Use this list to start your mind working about what will help keep you sane during what can be a pretty friggin' insane time.

A Staying Sane Primer— An Incomplete List If Ever There Were One

- Rent or buy entire seasons of your favorite TV show, preferably a comedy, and watch them all. (Suggestions: *Arrested Development, Scrubs*)

- Watch the Food Network. Planet Cancer member WhyNotMe points out the irony here: "I could hardly think of anything that sounded good to eat, nor could I stand the smell of most foods during chemo, yet I believe I watched the Food Network almost ten hours a day. There was something comforting about the shows."

- Buy yourself treats online. They don't have to be expensive, but the anticipation alone is worthwhile if you're cooped up indoors. This exercise is also a helpful gauge of how whacked out on Ativan you are during treatment. Says Denny: "I bought something from Nascar.com, which I assume was a shirt. It was done while heavily drugged, and now I'm on their mailing list forever."

- Look up restaurant menus on the Internet, and imagine eating there.

- Watch the Travel Channel.

- Virtually roam around the globe via Google Earth. Imagine you're being flown around on a magic carpet named Percocet. Visit the Eiffel Tower, the pyramids, and the Great Wall of China—in one evening!

- Video games (try online games that allow you to chat with others).

- Exercise. Walk up and down your driveway, around the block, whatever works for your energy level. Also, the Nintendo Wii offers exercise-centric video games.

- Go to movies. (It's fine to go by yourself!)

- Read novels, write snail-mail letters, and revive the past millennium!

- Volunteer. Sometimes helping others is the best way to get out of your own head. Depending on your energy level and the state of your immune system, you can do anything from taking donations at the food bank, to fostering kitty cats, to tutoring in an after-school program.

Also, it's worth mentioning again not to forget to laugh at the more than infrequent absurdity on this Planet. This dispatch is a great example:

So, I'm scurrying back from the coffee shop at my hospital trying to make my appointment on time, and I pass an office marked, and I'm not kidding here, "Tumor Registry." I stopped. Looked again. Surely I read that wrong. Nope. "Tumor Registry." Now, I have to believe that this has some kind of serious and useful function, but you can imagine where my brain went.

"Um . . . yes. I'd like something small and benign, preferably away from any vital organs. Do they come in fashion colors? I'm on kind of a lavender kick lately." Seriously?! Maybe they have different tumors on display and you can just scan them with your own little scanner gun? Clubb Cancerr at Target. "Beep. Yes. I'd like a set of three. Enter."

Or maybe you're shopping for a friend? "Do you gift wrap? How about shipping out of state? I'd like the card to read, 'Congrats on your ovarian mass. Now you can throw away all of your tampons! Kiss. Kiss. Christine.'"

And here's an idea. "What is your return policy? I have a twenty-one-centimeter Krukenberg tumor I'd like to return. Yes, it was really giving me trouble with bladder function, not to mention the unsightly bulge. No cash value, huh? Well can I get hospital credit? Apply it toward my chemo and CT scans."

Yep. The mind reels. So, I'm standing there in front of this office giggling uncontrollably. I'm totally cracking myself up and really want to share this with someone, but then it occurs to me that almost no one is going to find this funny but me. I should have taken a cell phone pic. Maybe next time.

—CHRISTINE BLUMER

Christine's hilarious dispatch notwithstanding, cancer registries do serve an important purpose on the Planet. In each state, hospitals and other treatment facilities report data to the state registry about tumor incidence, type, stage, treatment, etc. The Centers for Disease Control and Prevention (CDC) oversee the National Program of Cancer Registries (NPCR), which collects info from the states. This comprehensive data complements that collected by the National Cancer Institute's Surveillance, Epidemiology, and End Results (SEER) registry program. The two programs use the data they collect to evaluate risk-related behaviors and environmental risk factors, to illuminate the most effective screening and monitoring practices and to target the best research being done for certain cancers. We don't know their interstate shipping policy.

Exercise

Truly, when I'm exercising I forget about cancer a little bit—it makes me feel strong and kind of like my body is not giving up on me. Exercise makes you feel better overall. I don't think I could live without it.

—BEVERLY

For years, exercise has been viewed as somehow optional or even counterproductive to cancer treatment. You're diagnosed and it's all about getting through treatment—the active things you can't do anymore slide off the radar, and nobody's telling you what should replace, say, a full-court game of hoops or running three miles.

Don't slip into the couch potato vortex! Mountains of studies correlate exercise with improved tolerance for treatment, improved recovery, and reduced recurrence. It's not only good for your emotional state; when done correctly, exercise can also:

- Speed recovery from treatment

- Help your body heal

- Help boost your immune system

- Reduce nausea and fatigue

- Increase energy levels

- Play an important role in preventing other diseases

- Prevent the recurrence of many types of cancer

For the general population, the American Cancer Society recommends thirty minutes of physical activity per day to receive health benefits, although any kind of movement for any length of time is good. These things have all been proven again and again. Exercise should be a top priority for anyone diagnosed with cancer!

The biggest challenge can be figuring out how to exercise. It's hard to say, exactly, but just take some time to assess where you are—physically and mentally—and get started on something that feels comfortable to you. *Note:* Now is not the time to start training for a marathon if you've never run more than a mile. Think about what you like to do and what you are physically capable of.

Remember that both cardiovascular exercise and resistance training can be beneficial to cancer survivors. Both types of exercise affect different systems in your body in important ways. Cardiovascular exercise helps your circulatory systems; resistance training strengthens your bones and positively impacts your endocrine system, which regulates your hormones. Are you drinking the Kool-Aid yet? Read on for some specific pointers about exercising your cancerous butt.

{ How to Exercise with Cancer }

by Ethan Zohn

"Hey, I think I just killed myself. Don't worry, some wizard in the gym caught me," I said. After a long, frantic, muffled, sweaty, chemo-induced pause, I continued: "Does Harry Potter belong to my gym?"

That was the voice mail I left my girlfriend, Jenna, when I accidentally pushed myself too hard and passed out cold. I don't even remember making the call. This was a simple but important lesson. No matter how much I wanted to, I couldn't handle the same intensity of workouts I was doing before I started treatment.

Ever since my older brothers invented the games "Kick the soccer ball at baby E's head" and "Chase Chubb-E until he cries," exercise has been a huge part of my life. Working out is what I love. It's my safe space, my escape from the real world. I played sports growing up and ended up playing pro soccer for six years all over the world. I was actually training for a marathon when I got diagnosed with Hodgkin's disease.

The way chemotherapy affected me wasn't unlike running a marathon. In a marathon, as time goes on and the miles build up, the harder it is on

There are potential cardiac effects with radiation and some chemo drugs, such as Adriamycin. Heart complications are usually only seen above a certain cumulative dose, but there are some subclinical effects at lower doses. Although this is probably not an issue for gentle exercising, check with your oncologist before getting your heart pumping too fast.

your body and the worse you feel. But when it's over, the runner's high sets in and a huge sense of accomplishment pulses through your veins. Same with chemo. At first I was shocked at how energetic and strong I was feeling. But after a month, it became a royal pain in the ass, literally and figuratively. Eight minutes on the treadmill and I was sucking air like a beached fish. Impossible! Two sets of bicep curls and my arms felt like Play-Doh. My whole body, though it appeared OK, was a hot useless mess on the inside. I felt embarrassed, depressed, and unmotivated. So I stopped working out completely.

Bad decision. There are some very dark days going through chemotherapy. Everything is failing. You can't eat. You feel miserable. You have no energy. But you've got to be able to mentally, emotionally, and spiritually get through that. I realized that the human body can endure a lot of mistreatment; it's the mind that is truly fragile. So, I drew from the physical and mental conditioning I developed as an athlete. I dug deep and used the pieces of me that felt scared, that were angry and powerless.

After about two weeks of sloth and self-pity, I went back into the gym. I wanted to own my can-

cer. I would make it my bitch. I got off the couch, promptly overdid it, and left my girlfriend a bizarre voice mail that mentioned a kid wizard.

After Harry Potter thwarted my near-death experience, I made a conscious decision to cut back a little and just enjoy the process of working out. I didn't need to whale on my pecs, get my heart rate to 200, or squat until my quads exploded. During chemotherapy and radiation, about 70 percent of patients have fatigue and loss of energy. Too much rest may result in loss of function, strength, and range of motion. Do as much as you can, but as chemo continues, be prepared to tailor your exercise regime. Reduce intensity, drop weight, jog slower, cut back on reps.

Every day during treatment I tried to get some form of exercise. My favorite workout plan was a long brisk walk from my couch to Jamba Juice for a smoothie. Far from a marathon, but there *is* a smoothie at the finish line. At least I forced myself outside, got my legs moving and my heart pumping. It's important to break the cycle and to establish a routine. Research has linked regular exercise to reduced fatigue and to being able to do normal daily activities without major limitations, thus improving one's quality of life. Which is what you want during this crappy time.

Cancer touches you in every way: mental, physical, social, spiritual, environmental. Every day I looked forward to getting out of bed and hitting the gym for some light weights or a session on the stationary bike. These little efforts were a big departure from what I was used to, but it made sense: Toward the end I was at about 25 percent of full physical capability. I felt better working out under this lighter plan. Yoga and stretching helped me focus and de-stress; maybe your key activity is also yoga. Or working in the garden. Or

{ **My persistence in exercising, even if it's just a walk to Jamba Juice, has served me well in enduring the toxic body-blow that is chemo.** }

jujitsu. Get it? Anything safe, effective, and enjoyable is the best choice for exercising during cancer treatment.

Sometimes I split my workout into three twenty-minute sessions and hit the gym two or three times a day. I'd walk in the a.m., do one set each of chest, biceps, triceps, back, legs, shoulders, and calves after lunch, and then, at night, do some stretching and yoga. It broke up the monotony of the day and gave me something to look forward to. Even if I did nothing, at least I "worked out three times." (See how awesome that sounds? Despite having cancer, you worked out three times in one day!)

Also, if I was having sleeping problems—another side effect—exercise tired me out a bit and got me relaxed and able to sleep a little better. Don't get me wrong. There were days I felt so miserable, depressed, and lazy I couldn't do anything. I felt more like a walrus trapped on my couch than a former pro athlete. I didn't even

enjoy watching *Seinfeld;* now that's serious. But the thought of not exercising would make me feel worse. It helped psychologically to move and free myself from the constraints of cancer. I'm not long out of treatment now and I'm probably at 50 percent physically. I go back for some tests in a month, and I might have to have more treatment. I'm picking up my reps and distances correspondingly, but not overambitiously.

Here's what I know: My persistence in exercising, even if it's just a walk to Jamba Juice, has served me well in enduring the toxic body-blow that is chemo, and it will continue to serve me well in fighting this crazy-ass disease.

If you're looking for an easy way to start a home workout routine, look no further than your iPod. You can quickly and easily download your whole exercise routine on your iPod and take it absolutely anywhere. It's like having a personal trainer in your back pocket. You can find downloadable programs by Googling "iPod workouts."

Also remember that the Nintendo Wii has good exercise programs, including yoga! Play an active game of tennis, bowl several frames, or crack some home runs in baseball. You can work up a sweat on Wii.

Guides to the Planet

After winning *Survivor: Africa,* Ethan Zohn cofounded Grassroot Soccer, an international organization that uses Africa's most powerful role models, pro soccer players, to educate youth about the dangers of HIV/AIDS. He also created Grassroot Soccer UNITED, a U.S.-based awareness campaign, and dribbled a soccer ball 550 miles from Boston to Washington, D.C. In May 2009, Ethan was diagnosed with a rare form of Hodgkin's lymphoma called CD20+ Hodgkin's lymphoma. After battling this for six months, the cancer returned; he completed an autologous stem cell transplant and got his first clean scan while this book was being completed. Ethan is an ambassador for Stand Up to Cancer and the national spokesman for America Scores. Ethan also keeps himself busy working with multiple charity organizations, including the LIVE**STRONG** Foundation, Colon Cancer Alliance, Autism Speaks, and PETA. Currently Ethan hosts *Earth Tripping,* an eco-friendly travel adventure show. Ethan returned to reality TV as a contestant on *Survivor All-Star, Fear Factor,* and

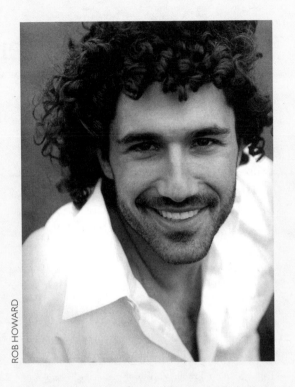

ROB HOWARD

Eco-Challenge, and he hosted two soccer television shows, the *MSG Soccer Report* and *F.C. Fox.* He was featured in the documentary film *A Closer Walk* along with the Dalai Lama, Bono, and Kofi Annan. Ethan has also starred in commercials for Nike and Hewlett-Packard, hosted MTV specials, and reported from the sidelines of Major League Soccer games.

Exercise and Cancer, Part Deux

by Marion Cimbala

Eighteen days after I was diagnosed, I wrote: "Tuesday morning I dragged my whiny self off the couch and met a friend at the pool to kickboard and talk. We kicked laps and talked about, among other things, her grandmother, who had refused bacon and eggs at the hospital through the last days of her life because she was concerned it might raise her cholesterol. Her cholesterol really didn't matter—she was dying anyway—but she stuck to her beliefs right to the end.

"After my friend left, I stayed and swam a few laps and I realized how amazingly wonderful it felt to swim. I don't think it has ever felt better than it did that morning. I realized how lucky I was to still feel good enough to swim. I thought about her grandmother, and how important it is to keep doing the things we love to do with our lives, and how we have a choice to keep believing in what we believe in no matter what is going on around us.

"So, as I swam along, feeling strong and alive, it became very clear to me that I may have cancer, but cancer does not have me. It just doesn't."

During and after surgery I was not able to swim for a few months so I went to the gym and walked like a senior citizen—very, very slowly on a treadmill. There was no one to ask for specific advice, so I worked cautiously in the months following my treatment. I felt very fragile, but I realized that the only way I was not going to feel fragile was to get moving.

It worked. A few months later I started feeling good again.

Almost a year later I was doing some core exercises, feeling really strong and pushing myself as I had pre-cancer. Unfortunately no one in the oncology world mentioned to me that removing all of my abdominal lymph nodes had left me vulnerable to lymphedema. I had never heard of lymphedema, a possible by-product of your lymph system being compromised by surgery, radiation, or another form of treatment; in lymphedema, lymph fluid accumulates somewhere in your body, which results in painful swelling and the potential for infections. It's chronic, and you can treat it, but there's no cure. I found out about lymphedema after it was too late, and I'll have this swelling in my legs for the rest of my life. To avoid lymphedema, consult with your doc to learn if your lymph system as been compromised in any way via treatment or surgery; with that knowledge you can create the right exercise plan. (It's very important to note that exercise does not cause lymphedema: Actually, because movement and exercise help move fluids through your system, exercise in moderation actually helps prevent lymphedema.) Your watchword should be "moderation."

If you aren't currently exercising, start by walking, stretching, and lifting things you have around your house as if they're weights. (There is absolutely nothing wrong with using a bottle of wine to do curls and presses before you drink it!)

If you are currently fit, stay with it, but know that you'll most likely have to modify your routine at some point during treatment. The simplest way to gauge your effort is to use a RPE scale (rating of perceived exertion). On a scale of one to ten, one is a slow walk, and ten is a mountain stage in the Tour de France. During treatment or if you are not currently very fit, your best bet is to keep your exertion level at about a four because you want to support your immune system without stressing it. After treatment is over, you can start moving the exertion up using interval training (e.g., move your effort up to level six or seven for periods of twenty seconds to five minutes).

Guides to the Planet

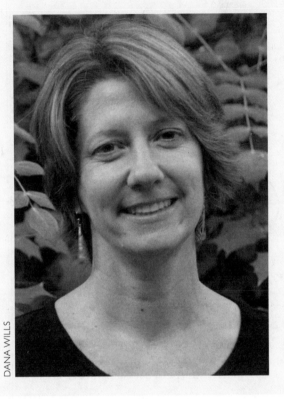

DANA WILLS

Six years ago after spending fifteen years in Austin, Texas, working in sports injury rehabilitation, event planning, and volunteering for numerous community causes, Marion Cimbala was diagnosed with cancer. After treatment (and the simultaneous adoption of her now five-year-old son), she became dedicated to improving the lives of people dealing with cancer. She continues to raise money and awareness through organizing large events, advocates for cancer funding at the city, state, and national levels, and has founded an organization to provide exercise and rehabilitative services to survivors. Marion also consults with dozens of nonprofit agencies to improve the care and services that people receive.

Nutrition

Nutrition and cancer care can be a scary trap. I feel that anything that makes you feel guilty cannot be good for you. The best advice I ever got was from a Chinese acupuncturist whom I asked for a good cancer diet. He had three words: "variety and moderation."

—KAIROL ROSENTHAL

No way will I stop drinking coffee. I'm here to enjoy everything I can.

—RILEYJAZZ

The best word to describe the volume and content of available information about cancer and nutrition is "minefield." A quick Google search for those two words together brings up more than forty-two *million* results. Yikes. We'll *all* be dead by the time we try to sift through that. And

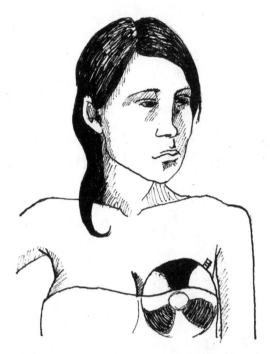

Top 9 Things You Would Rather Not Hear from Your Physician

True stories from members of the Young Survival Coalition,
which serves young women under forty with breast cancer.

9. When complaining to my plastic surgeon about the funky shape of my tissue expander, he said, "Well, it's sort of like a beach toy that is not fully inflated yet."

8. When asked to take part in a clinical trial suitable for Stage II cancer, I asked my oncologist, "So that means I'm Stage II, then?" And he replied, "Yeah, at least!"

7. After taking samples of my tumor, my physician asked, "Do you want to see them? They look like little tiny pieces of angel hair pasta."

6. After discussing plastic surgery for breast cancer, my plastic surgeon said, "You know they are never going to look real."

5. When discussing with my oncologist about getting my port removed, he said, "Well, I guess we can put it back in if we need it."

4. My oncologist said, "Well, everything is fine—for now."

3. My primary oncologist asked me, "So, who is your primary oncologist?"

2. My plastic surgeon remarked, "I hate making nipples."

1. Arriving to get a mammogram a few years after a breast cancer diagnosis, he says, "So, why are you here?"

how is it possible to determine who, out of all those millions of confident postings, speaks the truth that is right for you?

The other thing about food is . . . well, it can be a really loaded topic because we have a lot of emotional attachments to food. What we eat, when we eat, who we eat with, what our moms said to us about dessert when we were six—all of these things play into how we regard food and how we feel about ourselves when we eat. Food is a critical component of our health and well-being, but it's also important to feel good about what you are eating.

If you take a spoonful of guilt or resentment with every bite you put in your mouth, it's *not helping*. So listen to your body and serve up a generous bowlful of common sense and appreciation, along with food that will strengthen and nourish your body while providing enjoyment and pleasure at the same time.

{ Food Is Power }

by Lena Huang
nutrition and fitness editor, CURE *magazine*

Whether you are recently diagnosed or a survivor, it's hard not to feel out of control once you've had cancer. Some strange monster entered your body, made a home, controlled your destiny, and maybe still does. It sent you on a mind-bending roller-coaster ride of emotions, sacrificed your body, and made everyone who loves you feel helpless. And maybe it stole things from you never to be replaced: a beautiful mane of hair, high school graduation, a dream job.

But one of the most important things you can do is to take back your life, and one way you can do that is through good nutrition. Food is power. Food heals. Good nutrition provides the building blocks for a healthy immune system, a strong heart and mind, solid bones and muscles. It gives you energy when you are feeling low. And especially for cancer patients, it helps repair tissue damaged by surgery and/or chemotherapy. It helps you fight that monster.

But before you do a total purge of your pantry, keep in mind some key points:

- No one food is going to cure cancer. No, it's not the acai berry, gingko, or grandma's secret concoction. Stay with what we know about balanced diets. Eat more fruits, vegetables, and whole grains. Choose lean proteins, such as fish and beans, and limit your intake of red meat and processed foods. Stay away from items high in saturated fats, trans fats, salt, and sugar.

- Your dietary plan needs to be personalized for you. If you are on chemotherapy, some things are known to interfere, such as green tea with the drug Velcade (bortezomib). If you have neutropenia, your weakened immune system needs to be protected from bacteria, so those fresh fruits and veggies need to be cooked.

- Mouth sores or difficulty swallowing may make eating a challenge as well. Your doctor, nurse, or dietitian can help you determine what you should eat or not eat based on your individual situation.

- Supplements and antioxidants also need to be approved by your doctor, nurse, or dietitian. Some supplements and antioxidants, especially taken in higher doses than the recommended daily allowance, interfere with chemotherapies and reduce their anticancer effects.

- You are what you eat, so love your body and treat it well.

As CURE's nutrition/fitness editor, I have interviewed many health experts on the importance of nutrition during the cancer journey. Across the board, these experts agree that good nutrition is like good medicine. In 2008, I interviewed Barrie Cassileth, Ph.D., chief of the integrative medicine service at Memorial Sloan-Kettering Cancer Center in New York, and I think she summarized it best: "No diet can cure cancer, but eating a balanced diet sufficient in proteins, vitamins, and minerals gained through foods—not through supplements—is the best treatment for everyone, whether you have cancer or not, to keep your body strong."

Food Tips from Lena's Nutrition Desk at Cure Magazine

While there are many ways to eat healthy, here are a few tips to eat better:

- When you are out, **ask for more healthful options** and don't be shy. Most restaurants are willing to accommodate switching fried chicken for grilled or a salad for fries.

- **Keep fresh fruit on the counter** or on a shelf in the refrigerator where you can see it to remind you of better snack options. An apple or orange gives you energy, vitamins, and fiber. If you have a choice, choose the fruit over the juice.

- **Add color and nutrition to your meal** by including shredded carrots, zucchini, or similar vegetables on a green salad, in casseroles, in burritos, or in just about anything. This is an easy way to increase your daily intake of veggies and to add more nutrients to your meals.

- **Eat more whole grains** by choosing whole grain bread for your sandwiches, trying brown rice or whole wheat pasta, and using rolled oats or crushed whole grain cereal to bread chicken or fish, or to add in meat loaf.

- **Become a locavore!** Eat local by growing your own food, checking out a farmers' market, or asking your grocer for locally grown foods. Not only do local foods taste better because they are fresher, you are also helping the environment by not supporting shipped foods, for which fuel must be burned to transport.

There are also many resources to help you eat better. Always check out www.curetoday.com for the latest cancer information, but if you want some basic food information, check out the U.S. Department of Agriculture's Web site at www. mypyramid.gov, which introduces the new food pyramid, offers a personalized dietary plan, and has educational resources.

A registered dietitian is also a wonderful resource that many hospitals and cancer centers offer free of charge. A dietitian can help you make healthier food choices and also offer aid if you have special food challenges, such as mouth sores, or have side effects impacted by food, such as diarrhea. You can also find a dietitian certified to work with cancer patients and survivors through the American Dietetic Association at www.eatright.org. The American Cancer Society has a wealth of information on eating before, during, and after cancer at www.cancer .org, and sells cookbooks as well.

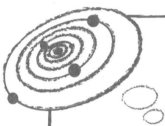

Dispatches
from the Planet

Because I started reading a lot of diet-related materials, on- and offline, I was increasingly drawn toward wine—particularly red and its supposed health benefits. (To my mode of thinking, if I was going to drink anyway, why not drink something that might also offer some potential benefits?) One night pretreatment anxiety got the better of me. I popped open a bottle of merlot … and didn't stop till the whole thing was gone. (By the end, my wife explained, I vehemently lamented the fact that they were "making the bottles smaller these days.")

I also seem to recall something about praising unrepentant old drunks—in this case, Peter O'Toole, I believe; I'd just read an interview with him in which he had basically said that, in spite of his own poor health and the passing of many of his contemporaries due to alcohol use and abuse, he'd do it all over again the exact same way given the chance. (Somewhere around the time the bottle got "too small," I told my wife that I was going to be the "Peter O'Toole of chemotherapy.")

—William Patrick Tandy

> **Mixing alcohol with certain chemo drugs can be really bad—for example, sometimes it can cause severe drug hepatitis. Talk to your doc if you're thinking about getting your drink on.**

{ Just Juice It }

by Cody Wilshire

Coming from a very Mediterranean family, and growing up in the Mediterranean, I have always known, understood, and loved the natural goodness of a Mediterranean diet. A diet that focuses mostly on vegetables, lean protein, and healthy fats, it's been touted as one of the healthiest in the world. Every doctor I've ever had has always complimented me on being such a great eater, on being so healthy, so well-educated, so focused on nutrition. If everything was so great, then why, when I ate this way, did I feel so awful?

I always listen to my body, something that isn't really easy at times, and I decided to delve into a bit of research. I always tell people that if you truly, honestly want to know something, then you will stop at nothing to educate yourself on it. So I took my own advice. I did research. Google became my second form of education; the bookstore became my best friend.

From the research I found and the knowledge I gained, I kept finding myself coming back to the same thing: raw eating, natural detoxing. . . . Chlorophyll, chlorophyll, chlorophyll! I started juicing green vegetables and drinking them every morning (a combination of cucumber, celery, kale, lemon, and sprouts). It was harsh on my stomach at first, but I found my energy skyrocketing. Each week I'd add more raw foods to my daily diet (lots of different types of salads and wraps, sandwiches and green smoothies).

I found my body responding better to treatment and to everyday situations, whether they were cancer-related or not. My body felt "clean" and healthy. I immersed myself in more books and all the knowledge on "living foods" or "raw eating" that I could. I decided to stick with what is called an 80/20 diet—80 percent of the food I consume daily is raw; 20 percent is cooked. The 20 percent flexibility allowed me to not feel as restricted, and sprouted grain bread is a savior when you're undergoing treatment.

I won't lie: Some days it was difficult to stick with the juicing. With chemotherapy being so toxic, every day my body would detox as if it were the first day again, because it was. But it was worth it: My body feels so balanced and strong when I stick to it—how could I deny that?

I wish I could say that I'm cured now, that I'm no longer undergoing treatment, that this diet "cured" my cancer, but I can't. What I can say is that every time I see my doctors they are surprised by my energy, by my "glow," by how great I am feeling both inside and out. To this day, the first thing I do every morning is make my "green lemonade" (juiced green vegetables with lemon) and to this day, every time I do, I swear its energizing effect is three times more intense than the cups of espresso I used to drink every morning.

Cancer or not, this diet is something I'll stick with for the rest of my life. It's so simple and so earth-shattering at the same time, it completely revolutionized my world. And it all started with just listening to my own body and a fun little Google search for "cancer, diet, help."

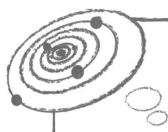

Dispatches
from the Planet

Here are a few more suggestions of things that worked for a fellow Planet native during treatment.

1. Intravenous vitamin infusion (mainly C with some other vitamins mixed in). This was the most awesome response I ever had. If I felt like I was close to death, vitamin C infusion is the first on my list. It was amazing!

2. Grapefruit juice daily cured my upset stomach problems and seemed to make me feel better.

3. Changing my diet. I went from eating greasy fast food, Cokes, chocolate, and junk food to a more natural diet of fruits and veggies and smaller amounts of meat. Between this and the grapefruit juice, my acid reflux went way down.

4. Vitamin supplements. I was extremely anemic and low on iron, so I took extra iron, magnesium, potassium, a small amount of calcium to get correct magnesium/calcium balance, vitamin A, zinc, and E.

5. During chemo I drank something called Hippocrates soup made into a drinkable mush. It was the first thing I was able to drink after about three to four days of not eating anything. Boy, does it give you good energy quickly.

6. I did a couple of other things like the parasite cleanse and the liver flush, and I don't know if it helped my body battle the cancer, but I was amazed.

—Sherri

Hippocrates soup, some say, derives from the man himself. Its health benefits are touted by many. Cook some up and be your own judge! One plus: The recipe doesn't require peeling any ingredients, so it's easier than you might think. Find the copyrighted recipe online.

Sex

I always had a very strong sex drive. You know, daily or more often. Now, it is all I can do to even consider it once a month. My husband is very supportive and all that, but that isn't the point. The point is I am incredibly frustrated at how my body is betraying me like this. Even if I do manage to get into it at all, the hot flashes and dryness ruin it. Does this last forever? I get so depressed by this. I went to the pharmacy section to browse the KY aisle, and just started bawling, right there in the grocery store.

*—*Rachael

As far as how long it has been, I won't even say, but Dubbya's first term wasn't over. I liken it to

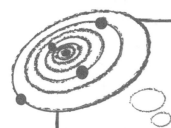

Dispatches from the Planet

Actual intercourse would be great, but if it can't happen, it can't happen. In my case it usually can't happen. Get it any way you can. That's what I think. Try anything. Even third-party products to help satisfy her. Trust me, I know it can be humiliating to have to resort to using a dildo on your wife. Trust me, I know! But I would try anything to make her feel like I care. I think that is a huge part of a man's responsibilities. Take care of her needs no matter what.

—superfluke

I started dating a new guy about six months before my diagnosis. I had to have a mastectomy and wasn't able to get immediate reconstruction. I didn't know if this relationship was even going to survive my road ahead. He proved to be a very supportive and loving person. It was very strange for me at first. After surgery, when we got intimate, I wouldn't even let him take my shirt off. After

I got comfortable with that, I wouldn't let him touch me. It felt really strange because of the sensory loss. Every once in a while I would get insecure about how he felt about me and my body. Even when I got reconstruction—and at that point we had been together two years—I still went through a similar thing. I wouldn't let him look at me. But things do get better over time.

—Jen

I can tell you that even though I was not directly hit with radiation down below, the emotional effects of cancer treatment, self-image, etc., definitely affected me when I started a sex life again. Most of it was in my own head; in fact the first time I really was sexual again, I had a G-tube sticking out of my stomach, which was so awkward for me. I had never felt self-conscious before, but it really played with my psyche.

—Denny

boxing with marshmallows. It is soft and sweet,
but you ain't stinging nothin' like a bee.

—WILLIE

Sex? You think we're kidding, don't you? Besides some mild fantasies about the hot anesthesiologist who wheeled you into surgery or run-of-the-mill nurse fetishism, sex is probably the last thing on your mind. That's completely understandable. Even if your sex organs are not directly affected by your disease, cancer treatment can impact sexuality indirectly through fatigue, pain, worry, hormonal changes, and body-image issues.

Physical, mental, and emotional stress are the cancer trifecta of libido-killers, but there are things you can do to put you back on the path to friskiness again. The first is to realize that the mind is the most powerful sexual organ and that taking the first step of talking about sexual concerns with your partner, doctor, or a counselor might just be the hardest part of resolving them.

A less common by-product of cancer is that it sets one's sexuality on overdrive. You're scared and lonely and looking for comfort, perhaps, or you're exercising control in one arena that you know you can. Without replacing your shrink, we'll just say that sex never really solves problems—or at least the sort of problems that cancer brings about. (Yes, there is the infamous thread on Planet Cancer's forum My Planet—http://myplanet.planetcancer.org/—full of anecdotal evidence about masturbation giving a boost to the ol' blood counts. We asked our docs and though they said there's nothing supporting these claims, we won't tell you not to do it!)

Top 10 Attractions at the "Michael Diaz Dream Cancer Center for Young Adults"

Because don't we all want a happy ending? It's nice to dream.
Loosely based on Michael's "Cancerland" blog from My Planet

10. Radiation laser tag.

9. No candy stripers—just strippers named Candy.

8. Try your luck at a basketball shooting game, only the rim is about a foot away. Face it: None of us has the strength to shoot a normal distance.

7. Win cool prizes, like, like . . . insurance coverage for another year! Keep the fucking stuffed animal.

6. Those mist things spray the med of your choice. (Imagine that. Now imagine that spraying Dilaudid. Hellz yeah.)

5. All nurses' stations double as full-service bars. Push your nurse call button and order whatever the hell you want.

4. Vincristine or [INSERT NAME OF YOUR CHEMO HERE] is called "motherfucker": "Hey, I don't want any more of that motherfucker."

3. When you're prepping for surgery, you don't use any anesthesia. You just have sex until you pass out.

2. Everything is a game. You know, if you need to vomit, we bring in people you hate so you can vomit on them. Or we can line up the vomiters and see whose vomit is most toxic.

1. And how about the section where they give out nice, sensual massages to anyone who wants one? And you get a happy ending!

{ Sexuality and Intimacy on Planet Cancer }

by Sage Bolte,
ABD, LCSW, OSW-C oncology counselor,
Life with Cancer

(Much of the information provided in this article originally appeared in "The Leukemia and Lymphoma Society's Fact Sheet on Sexuality and Intimacy," also written by Ms. Bolte.)

People crave interaction. We have the natural desire to be touched, hugged, caressed, and loved. Whether this is fulfilled in a partnership or by close friendships, most people desire close relationships that involve intimacy at some level. Sexuality is more than just the act of sex. Your sexual self is influenced by physical, psychological, social, emotional, and spiritual factors. It can include the way you view yourself as a sexual being, whom you are attracted to, your feelings of sensuality, and sexual functioning.

Cancer and its treatments can impact how a person feels about their sexual self beyond just sexual function and fertility; it can extend to intimate relationships, regardless of age, race, religion, or health.

Sexuality and intimacy are not life or death issues; even so, they are very real quality-of-life issues that should be adequately addressed in the context of cancer and treatment. Sexuality and intimacy are not typically the first issues to be brought up by the health-care team, but they deserve more attention. As with all side effects or symptoms, it is critical to communicate with your health-care team about your experience to ensure you receive the best care plan possible.

Professionals who might be able to best address your sexual health concerns as they relate to your cancer experience include your oncologist, urologist, endocrinologist, gynecologist, oncology-certified nurse, sex therapist, oncology social worker, and the Walgreens employee who knows where the lube is.

Questions to ask your health-care team:

- What are the ways that treatment may affect my ability to have sex? How long will these effects last?

- Can I have sex while on treatment? Are there precautions I should take? Is it ever not safe to have sex?

- How will/has this treatment or diagnosis affect/affected my fertility? What are my options?

- Who else can I speak with about this topic?

- (For hospitalized patients) Can you help me arrange some private time with my partner, as long as it doesn't interfere with my medical care? (Related question: Do you have a disco ball you can mount on the ceiling temporarily, and can you throw some Al Green on my iPod?)

- How can I improve the way I feel about myself?

Communicating with Your Partner

Often, a cancer diagnosis can impact communication between partners, and this is especially true with communication about sex. It is really important that both of you take the time to express your concerns and needs as they relate to your individual sexual health and your sexual and intimate health as a couple. This may mean that you need to get creative about how to stay connected if what worked for you before no longer works.

Some partners feel as though it may be perceived as selfish to have and/or express their sexual and intimate needs, or are afraid they may (physically) hurt their partner who is going through treatment if they are physically intimate. For example, the partner may be afraid to do something as simple as cuddling or kissing if the person undergoing treatment has had pain or mouth sores, out of fear of increasing this discomfort. Or, if there are surgical scars, they may be afraid that by touching them they will cause pain or emotional discomfort and it has nothing to do with attraction.

The person with cancer may perceive his or her partner's lack of physical or intimate approaches as indicating a lack of interest: "Maybe he or she isn't attracted to me or doesn't want to be with me anymore." This can lead to emotional and physical distance and a lot of misunderstandings between partners. Therefore it is critical that you both keep the lines of communication open and speak to a professional if those lines break down.

Vaginal Dryness and Erection, Arousal, or Orgasm Problems

It is not uncommon to experience vaginal dryness or erection, arousal, or orgasm difficulties after a diagnosis of cancer. These effects can be due to the various cancer treatments and the medications given to manage side effects. Sexual difficulties may also be a sign of depression or anxiety, which is addressed differently, but such difficulties may also be caused by the medications prescribed to improve your anxiety and depression.

Discuss your current medications with a trusted health-care provider to see if any could be decreasing your ability to perform sexually. If a medication you are taking has sexual side effects, discuss with your provider any possible alternatives with lesser or no sexual side effects.

FOR THE GUYS:

- Assistive devices such as an external penile vacuum pump may be helpful if you are experiencing weaker erections. You can order them online. You may also be able to get a prescription from a urologist or your oncologist.

- There are medications that assist with increasing a male's desire response as well as erectile function.

- If you are experiencing changes in your erection, discuss with your provider the possibility of having your hormone levels tested and address any medications that may be impacting your erectile function.

FOR THE GALS:

- Vaginal dryness can occur due to menopause, antidepressants, or other medications. Using over-the-counter water-based lubricants, such as K-Y, Replens, Astroglide, etc., can help with vaginal dryness and pain during sex caused by dryness.

- Vitamin-E oil can also be a healing aid that can be used to help with vaginal health. It's sticky, so it isn't always the best to use as a sexual lubricant.

- Women who have decreased orgasms can practice Kegel exercises: While contracting the vaginal muscles, practice counting slowly to three, relax, and repeat numerous times.

FOR BOTH:

- Discuss with your doctor the possibility of adding a medication or hormone therapy to help with sexual response (this would most likely not be an option for people with hormone-sensitive cancers, such as some types of breast cancer and prostate cancer).

- Heightening/warming creams (for the clitoris or penis) can be used to enhance sexual response and desire.

- Work closely with a gynecologist or a urologist.

- Smoking and drinking alcohol can also affect erection difficulties and lack of interest.

- Don't rush your time together as a couple (or with yourself), as you are getting to know your body and sexual response again.

- Sexual enhancement aid Web sites, such as pureromance.com, were developed with the cancer survivor in mind.

Concerns for Couples

Loss of sexual desire (libido) can be caused by physical and emotional difficulties, fatigue, change in social life, fear of pain or breathlessness, guilt, and anger. They are all common side effects of a cancer diagnosis, and they can have a negative effect on sexuality and intimacy.

What used to be your "normal" routine for both sexual and social activity may need to be assessed and altered. If you are most alert and experience the least symptoms in the morning, then adjust your schedule accordingly to allow time to do the things you love when you feel at your best. This will take compromise by both the partner and the person with cancer.

- Use of foreplay, massage, erotica, or assistive devices can also help encourage the libido and sexual response.

- If sexual intercourse is not possible, use other forms of sexual intimacy, such as hand-genital manipulation, caressing, cuddling, hand-holding, and just lying together naked.

- Many times a diagnosis of cancer can cause partners and patients alike to experience symptoms of depression. If you are unable to find enjoyment in any type of activities or interaction with friends, discuss your concerns with a counselor or your physician to rule out depression.

- Role reversal, when one person becomes the caregiver and the other becomes the cared for, can cause stress and tension in a relationship as well as internal individual stress. This is not uncommon for a person with cancer and his or her partner to experience. Recognizing the issue and seeking counseling to find ways that both people can feel validated and have some control over their daily lives are important.

Painful Sex

If you have noticed that sex or vaginal exams (here's hoping that those aren't the same thing in your case) are painful, you may be experiencing vaginal stenosis (shrinking of the vaginal canal) or vaginal atrophy (weakening of the pelvic floor muscles). These can be caused by early menopause or graft-versus-host disease (GVHD), or might simply be a side effect from treatment. It is important to address and assess these phenomena with your team. Vaginal dilators can be used to lightly stretch the pelvic floor muscles and, in conjunction with Kegel exercises, can also strengthen the pelvic floor muscles.

Intimacy for the Single Person

Remember, sexuality and intimacy aren't just about sex. Think of ways to connect with your friends and family meaningfully.

If you are interested in exploring your sexual response, start with self-pleasuring exercises to get to know your body again and what makes you feel good. It is critical for you to not only feel comfortable with being touched but to know what does and does not feel good sensually and sexually. You may find that you have areas on your body with heightened sensitivity, and it is important that you know this before you introduce a partner.

- Take time to reconnect with yourself and find enjoyment in activities or interactions with loved ones.

- Find a support group where you can talk with other young adults who are struggling with some of the same ups and downs that you are.

- Choose one friend to meet with once a week to maintain an intimate and supportive network.

- Recognize that not every part of you has changed from your cancer diagnosis! You have control over whom you choose to surround yourself with and how you choose to express yourself.

- Cancer is *part* of your story, not your whole story!

I have yet to find a piece of literature that says, "People with a chronic illness should not have desire for sexual intercourse or intimate relationships." So, recognize the "should"s and "shouldn't"s that might cloud your thoughts on your sexual and intimate relationships and then start pursuing and achieving your desires.

A Frank Discussion of Cancer-Affected Sex

by Anonymous

I'll cut to the chase: Everyone wants a good, even great, sex life but tends to avoid talking about it if there are problems. This is especially true if you're old enough to be having sex while young enough to avoid depiction in an ad for erectile dysfunction. For me and my husband, cancer and the side effects of treatment thrust themselves into our lives and stayed around long enough—more than a decade—to force us to learn some coping skills.

During a vital time when the connection between us needed to be the strongest—when he was depending on me to not only take care of him but also love him unconditionally, cancer and all—we were losing the sexual and sensual intimacy we previously shared. And in the midst of every other bodily function, the discussion about sex wasn't being encouraged or even acknowledged in our medical community. We were facing mortality along with the loss of an intimacy that should be greedily consumed—hell, taken for granted—by twenty- and thirtysomethings! Sexuality and intimacy don't always have to be affected by cancer (or at least affected any more than what results from having to juggle an additional huge stress in life), but they certainly can be, so it's best to be as prepared and open to discussion as possible.

With knowledge gained during our own years of trial and error as well as professional advice, I've put together what I consider the most valuable points. They are written from the perspective of a committed heterosexual partnership without children, but I hope they also resonate with those in other relationship scenarios.

Let's Talk . . . About Sex.
(In Case You Weren't Already
Channeling Salt-n-Pepa).

The phrase "we need to talk" is especially cringe-worthy when it's followed by "about sex." But for many cancer patients, their partners (if in a relationship), and their medical team, that's exactly what needs to happen—talk about sex and fertility. For example, a decrease in libido or change in sexual function could be either symptoms or side effects, so let your doctor know about them as you would any other notable change in habit or bodily function, and the sooner the better. Early on, ask what effects cancer and the treatment for cancer may have on your sexuality and fertility, and then revisit the topic frequently throughout your treatment. Once the subject is brought up and given appropriate consideration, it's easier to discuss and broach again if needed, from both the patient and provider sides. (And I've experienced the reverse to be true, also: If the topic is raised and inadequately addressed by the medical team or dismissed by the patient offhand, then it's less likely to be brought up again by either party.)

Speaking from experience, I know this isn't as easy as it sounds. I often walked a fine, tense line between pushing my husband into conversations he was reluctant or embarrassed to have and ignoring my own desire to help him and help us. We had to garner the nerve to (sometimes uncomfortably) continually bring up the topic with the oncologists because the specialists they had referred us to for tests all reported "normal" results and were done with the investigation, so everything should be working fine, right? Uhhhh—no. Come to find out, often it's the nurses who have more information and ideas for specific referrals to specialists, sex therapists, tests, or techniques; they are also often more approachable, more accustomed to, and even more often trained to field questions relating to sexuality.

Intimacy Overload

When living a life that includes cancer, you end up talking a lot about numbers, counts, scans, port-a-caths, neutropenic precautions, and input/output statistics, which are all intimate topics. However, sometimes it's difficult enough to even discuss physical sexual intimacy, much less do it. Our counselor once said that the two of us shared so many other intimate interactions aside from sensuality that there was already an overload that left no room for any other intimate things, like sex. That really made sense, but I had never thought of it in that way! There may not be many solutions for this cancer partner conundrum aside from bringing in an outside caregiver for the medical needs, which can be impractical or undesirable. However, simply recognizing this fact about intimacy overload went a long way to dealing with my frustration over lack of intimate sexual connection or communication about it, and also relieved me from some feelings of resentment over not being able to enjoy what were supposed to be my best sexual years as a newlywed, wife, and woman.

Image Isn't Everything
(Even Though It May Feel Like It)

Especially when cancer becomes a part of a newish but committed relationship, as it did in our situation, it was surely a test of many things, including compatibility, communication skills, trust, and patience. I was constantly reassuring him that he was handsome, attractive, and sexy (and not just to me, but overall). Unfortunately, well-deserved flattery did little to raise the self-image he had of a guy no longer able to work, work out at the gym, or even have the illusion of control over his life at times. He had a shaky new identity, one that he didn't ask for, didn't like, and didn't want to have to deal with the complications of. One of the last things on his mind was getting frisky, and I often felt like the nagging instigator. Rejection hurts each time, despite knowing there is love and caring underneath, and rejecting someone you'd, in a non-cancer world, want to be intimate with must feel awful too. Neither scenario is particularly bolstering to self-image. What I found most helpful was trying not to take repeated rejection personally, all the while encouraging my husband that I'd be there for him when he was ready.

In addition, I was increasingly feeling like a nurse (definitely not in a Naughty Nurse way) and stringently resisting the mothering role (definitely not sexy) I felt was descending upon my identity. Luckily, our amazing support system allowed us to take periodic breaks from this slippery slope, and his actual mom was enlisted to mother him! Novel solution, right? This resulted in his ability to finally relax into his dependence on someone who embraced that job, freed me to happily abdicate an uncomfortable role and, for a time, returned us to being simply best friends, spouses, and lovers again.

Bring Sensuality Back

Set aside however much time you have in your schedule (ten, twenty, thirty minutes) once a week to sit or lie down with your partner without the expectation or requirement of performing a sexual act. Take equal turns touching each other in various ways across every part of each other's bodies except the genitals. Do not initiate sex but allow yourselves to indulge in sensuality without pressure. If this brings up sexual urges in one or both, try to leave that for another time. (But, I get it—if it's been a loooong time and you really, really, really want to act on it, initiate sexual acts only if you both agree you'd like to proceed after the allotted time. However, be clear that the expectation of sex will not be looming in subsequent sensuality sessions.)

That Said, When the Time Is Right: Trying Is Important

Sometimes, as a cancer partner, I felt as though the effort was even more important than whatever resulted from it. If we tried and sex didn't work for whatever reason, whether it was physical or emotional, it could go either way: devastating and debilitating or worth the try, no matter the result. In the end, I always tried to encourage the effort. And, after all was said and done, my husband would agree he enjoyed our time together—the trying and connecting—despite the anticipatory worry and sometimes disappointment.

Use It or Lose It

Whatever euphemism you choose—keep the pipes clean, the chassis lubed, practice makes perfect—the expert we consulted agreed that the old adage is correct. Without regular reminders, the systems start to turn off, and it's even more

difficult to get back to whatever "normal" is, especially when contending with prior or continuing medical issues. That goes for both the diagnosed and the partner! If there isn't sexual interaction together, continue practicing on your own. Keep the communication open and, if possible, encourage each other to a little self-nurturing (yes, I'm talking about masturbation), and reassure one another that whenever the other is ready to return to "doing your own things" together, you will be eagerly waiting. That may be challenging since it requires a lot of patience and understanding on your part, but as long as you tend to yourself in the process, you'll hopefully be ready when your partner is again and not hold as much resentment that it took however long it did to happen.

No Expectations of the Body

Find a new way, or go back to a prior way, to be intimate that has no previous "only well body" reminders. My husband loved to have his forearm lightly scratched (and his butt cheeks, if I'm being completely honest). It may sound funny or juvenile but it felt soooooo good to him, and his body could still appreciate that pleasure. So, when I wanted to kiss or do more with him physically than he had the desire or ability to do, I would ask if it would be OK for me to lightly scratch his forearms. This worked really well in the hospital too. We bonded over that, and it was so heartening to see that the painful medical procedures that caused his nerves and body to flinch at the slightest touch hadn't affected his ability to still feel the pleasure of this intimacy I was experiencing with him.

Pull in a Pro

No, not that kind of pro. But there may come a time when you've been saying or trying the same things over and over without resolution and the two of you just aren't hearing each other anymore. There's a lot to be said for a fresh perspective, especially when it is from a medical professional such as a therapist, psychologist, psychiatrist, or sex therapist.

Fundamentally, my husband and I dealt with cancer-related challenges in different ways: He ignored the bad parts, waiting for a time when he could deal with them in a life without cancer, while I clung to the idea that, whatever the difficulty was, an attempt at improvement could be made in the meantime. I was often frustrated with his somewhat effective "denial" approach, and he resented me for pushing him at times. There was a vast disparity between approaches, but we loved each other and were committed to our relationship, and enlisting someone trained in the field helped us attempt to bridge that divide. After all, we were still alive and wanting to live our lives together to the fullest despite a cancer that would not relent.

Lastly, a Friendly Reminder

If you are engaging in sexual intimacy while your partner is receiving chemo—YAY!!! However, please remember to take precautionary measures to protect your partner's and your physical health, including using barrier methods of protection (condoms, dental dams). Yeah, yeah . . . seems logical now that I'm older, wiser, and not "in the heat of the moment," but I honestly didn't think of it at the beginning, and I consider myself to have a modicum of intelligence. A body clears out chemo and its toxicities through many fluids, functions, and mechanisms (doxorubicin pee, anyone?) including ejaculate and vaginal fluids, which may be damaging, especially to our delicate bits and pieces. So during sex and acts that expose you to each other's fluids, use precautions to take care of your partner and yourself.

Sex is life-affirming. It should be pleasurable. It's been proven to release endorphins, relieve stress, and even diminish the sensation of pain. And, if you think beyond the "chucka chucka bauw wauwww" to the point of procreation (even if that's not the goal or hope), it's actually "life" in action. As most discover at some point in their lives, especially when dealing with medical issues, sex is more than intercourse. Much more. And that can be an amazing aspect of a relationship when you've persevered through cancer, together.

Casualty

by Anonymous

I love this man
who thinks he's broken
inadequate
unable
from years of living
in a body of betrayal.

We try but the tugs
of war casually make a
casualty of sex despite talks
maneuvers
retreat
calling for a medic again
hoping to revive
in him what is held hostage
in me.

He doesn't know I flirt
with impropriety
with hope he'll surprise
leer
grope
caress
me awake.

Instead, I fondle his
pills into day after
day of the week
chart chemo
rads
trials
over weeks
months
years
not wanting to know when his last
bowel movement was.
But I do.

Instead, we talk about
we laugh at life
death
living
and that I want him to want
to want me
again.

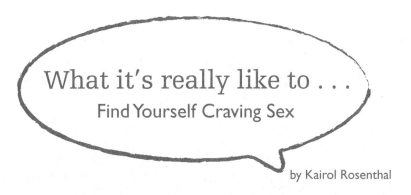

What it's really like to . . .
Find Yourself Craving Sex

by Kairol Rosenthal

My head still on the pillow, my eyes not yet open, the first conscious moment of my day always began with an insatiable desire to get laid. I was not a fifteen-year-old guy waking up with a puddle under the blankets. I was a twenty-seven-year-old woman with hormones wreaking havoc in my cancer-ridden body.

Calcium loss, hair loss, loss of appetite, heart palpitations, changes in libido. These were all side effects of my medication. There are trade-offs with most cancer treatments, and turning into a horndog was my price to pay. Considering that most patients in the cancer ward are puking their guts out or swimming in diarrhea, I was not going to complain. Instead, I simply decided to embrace my inner slut.

I had never been a prude, but like many women, for me doing the nasty had always been about more than sex; it was counterpart to my hope of finding love and connection. I had always been cautious, selective, scrutinizing before sleeping with a guy. But suddenly that was all gone. I was on a mission, and it was purely physical.

I lived in San Francisco and, though it was decades after the rise of Haight-Ashbury, the vibe of free love still lingered in the air. A year and a half into cancer, the number of men I slept with doubled. I felt no shame about my conquests. Cancer was enough of a drag without laying guilt

on top of it. I chose to look at this randy time in my life as a sociological study of what happens when a woman is just in it for the action.

I never had one-night stands. Instead most of these pseudo-relationships lasted for a few months at a time. I was forthright with these men about my cancer, and it did not take long for them to learn about my voracious appetite. Sometimes the tenor of these relationships was

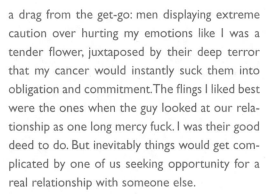

{ **I was on a mission,
and it was purely physical.** }

a drag from the get-go: men displaying extreme caution over hurting my emotions like I was a tender flower, juxtaposed by their deep terror that my cancer would instantly suck them into obligation and commitment. The flings I liked best were the ones when the guy looked at our relationship as one long mercy fuck. I was their good deed to do. But inevitably things would get complicated by one of us seeking opportunity for a real relationship with someone else.

Most of the time I was a fun, playful, wild little animal having the time of my life in order to counterbalance my fear of cancer. But when I was waiting for test results, suffering body aches, recovering from treatment, the raw human side of my cancer predicament met the raw animal side of my hormonal sex fest, and I would end up with these kind

yet unattached men holding me under the covers as I wept. Hormones or not, at heart I was a single woman who wanted deeply, and perhaps even more so because of my cancer, to be in love.

Fashion

Sometimes I think I can rock the fuzzy head and still look hot. Other times I feel like a sick-looking cancer patient.

—CANCERFREECANDY

You wake up one morning, and it hits you like a Mack truck. Not the fact of your own mortality, but the stench rising off the sweat suit you've been sporting around the hospital for the past four days.

Fashion is a priority for no one facing cancer, but there are ways around the standard southern-exposure hospital gowns and stained flannel pants from college. First, accept that comfort is key. After that, you just may feel better putting on fresh clothes every day. Clothes you won't be embarrassed to be seen in. Clothes that aren't so rank they could walk down to radiology by themselves.

Functional Treatment Attire

Repeat: You *don't* have to always wear the hospital gown they give you. If they insist, tell all medical staff they must pay the toll by mooning you before entering your room. Turnabout's fair play, after all. There are better-looking, more appropriate hospital gowns out there, so it doesn't hurt to research those alternatives if you like patterned cotton blends.

Try to keep metal out of your wardrobe so you can stay dressed for scans. That means no underwire bras, zippers, belts, Kevlar vests, etc. Depending on ports and other medical doo-

> **"Chemo chic"** (coined by HipiGuruPunk on Planet Cancer): A cancer-motivated appearance characterized by drastic weight loss, exfoliated skin, a professionally styled wig, and a lovely, radiation-inspired glow.

hickeys popping out of you, bras may not be an option anyway. Don't buy any new underthings until you have a grip on your new cancer bod and what you need to do to accommodate it.

Post-surgery, pants that can be pulled on are a must. More important, pants that can be pulled off quickly are a must. Talk to your surgeons about any postoperative restrictions you'll have, like not being able to reach over your head to pull on shirts or needing to keep body parts elevated. Cozy layers will keep you warm around the hospital and at home.

Ports and catheters in your chest will need easy access. It's a good idea to wear a button-front shirt when your catheter is being accessed and to run the tubing between a couple of the top buttons when you're getting hooked up to an IV. With T-shirts, the tubes have to either run all the way down your front and come out the bottom, or sprout up against your neck, neither of which is extremely comfortable and might pull or tug. And if, unthinking, you allow the catheter to be accessed from the top down while wearing a T-shirt, you're either going to be wearing that

T-shirt until the IV goes away, or you will be busting out the scissors to cut it off. So, just remember . . . a little forethought goes a long way.

Real-World Attire

When it's time to hit the world outside Linoleum Land, you may become a little more fashion-conscious. Decide if you want to cover your scars or show them off, and go shopping accordingly. Some people want to hide all traces of their disease by burying their chemo backpack under a sweater coat. Others flaunt the fanny pack bearing the pump and its associated tubing. Either way, go for it!

Sometimes it's a good idea to make things a little more obvious, to keep overzealous friends and near-strangers from squeezing a still-painful surgical site during an enthusiastic hug. Feel free to add accoutrements like slings and bandages to send a clear statement that you don't need to be manhandled at the moment.

Women especially have the wig vs. no wig debate, and there are good choices on either

> **Chemo backpack:** Sometimes people are on a constant chemo infusion over several days, and instead of keeping them in lockdown tied to an IV pole, they put the portable pump in a little fanny pack so they can walk around, go to class, work, etc. All while they're getting chemo. Ah, progress.

side. If you consider a wig, know that there are resources to find a good one at an affordable price. The wig's downside, however, is that it is hot and itchy. Many cancer-fighters scoff at adding one more element of discomfort to the list, so they turn to scarves and hats, or just keep it bare. You can mix it up, too, so don't feel as though you have to make one and only one decision. If losing your hair does end up making you feel less feminine, don't forget the addition of earrings, cute shoes, or comfy cotton dresses to remind you that you are still damn fine. OK?

{ Style during Treatment, from a Fashion Designer-Slash-Survivor }

by Kaylin Marie Andres

Cancer is so last year, darling.

I have always expressed myself by what I wear. From age five, when I'd pair pink Minnie Mouse shirts with floral and checkered leggings (oh, the horror), to now, I've always treated the street like a stage, dressing up for my grand ovation. I am a hopeless introvert, so fashion has always been

the best medium to express myself, enabling me to say something without uttering a word. This is one reason I decided to move to San Francisco and study design.

I was diagnosed with cancer a week before I was to start my senior year and finally design my thesis collection. I had just parlayed an internship into a full-time junior design position and had finished producing a fashion show for my own line, Sweet Marie. My life was just beginning when I got the devastating news that I'd have to move back in with my parents and start a grueling fourteen cycles of chemo and radiation. Fashion, which had been in the forefront of my life for as long as I could remember, was now taking a backseat to a deadly disease.

As I began treatment, my stage reverted to drab city streets. All I wanted to do was hide from the world. Quirky vintage dresses and heels were

> It's the superfluous details that we must hold onto in order to retain some level of normalcy through the hell that is cancer treatment.

replaced with sweats and hospital gowns, the uniform of the indisposed. Clothing once allowed me to express my individuality, but the hospital gowns I was forced to wear felt like inmate jumpsuits, stale gray and demoralizing.

I livened things up by buying dancewear in my favorite colors and soft cotton separates from American Apparel. I scoured eBay for vintage silk Hermès scarves for my baldy head. I kept some of my old dresses unpacked so on the rare day that I was feeling energetic, I could dress myself to the nines and feel "normal" again. All of these things helped profusely to keep my morale up.

Occasionally I would get fed up with feeling

like a (and I despise this term) "cancer victim." My hair fell out, my hormones stopped, I lost my curves. I felt alien. Dressing in my old clothing and a wig made me feel as though I had regained some of my lost femininity. One night, after weeks of recovering from chemo, I decided to dress up and meet friends at a bar in San Francisco. A man came up to me and, pointing to the lady with a shaved head in the corner, exclaimed, "Why do girls do that? It's so ugly!" He was using this woman's hairdo as a pickup line, hoping I'd chime in and agree. Maybe we'd have a laugh. I smiled sweetly and slowly lifted up my wig, revealing my hairless head. "Cancer," I replied. His horrified expression as he hurried away still brings a smile to my face.

Chemo eventually gave me neuropathy in my feet that made walking extremely painful. I was devastated at the thought of never being able to wear my precious shoe collection again. My mom had to buy comfort shoes for me to get around in—terribly tacky mules with rubber soles and faux fur lining. Granted, yes, they were comfy, but they looked like running-shoe roadkill. I've had nightmares about those abominations. But I digress. The neuropathy eventually went away, and the shoes along with it.

If all of this talk of fashion and footwear sounds trivial, well, you're right. It is. But it's the superfluous details that we must hold onto in order to retain some level of normalcy through the hell that is cancer treatment. Fashion reaffirms our identity in a time of crisis. Don't be embarrassed for missing your heels, your hair, and your fabulous style. It's part of what makes you you, and you will get to express yourself once more after treatment is over. I am, and it feels amazing to be on center stage again.

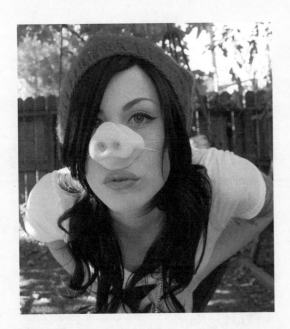

Guides to the Planet

Kaylin Marie Andres is a fashion designer and blogger based in San Francisco, California. She was diagnosed with Ewing's sarcoma in her pelvis at age twenty-three and went through eight months of chemo and adjunctive radiation. Her blog, Cancer Is Hilarious, candidly documents her experiences as a young adult living with a life-threatening disease. Check it out at www.cancerisnotfunny .blogspot.com. Kaylin is also designing a treatment-friendly and (yes) cancer-inspired collection—check out some of her designs and monitor the collection's progess at www.hellosweetmarie.com.

{ Style Icons for Completely Bald White Guys }

by Curtis Luciani

If you're a Caucasian male—and particularly if your natural skin tone is on the "pasty" end of the spectrum—you may find it difficult to confidently sport the hairless dome that chemotherapy leaves you with. I know I did. After my hair fell out, I discovered that I had a nice, smooth skull—quite a relief—but that relief was overtaken by concern that I looked like an out-of-shape neo-Nazi.

Completely bald white guys don't tend to be fashion icons, but an august few have pulled off the look with panache. If you're having trouble finding the right style to accompany your newly shiny head, here are some guys worthy of emulation. Following their example may make you the sharpest dude at your local infusion clinic:

The Delicate Artist (Michael Stipe of R.E.M.): This alt-rocker's contemporary look is perfect for frail fellows with poetic spirits. The rumpled suit says, "I'm an artist, so I like to show some grace, but I'm also kind of a mess . . . because I'm an artist." And then sneakers add a dash of cheek and comfort. (Contemporary Stipe is not to be confused with early '90s Stipe, with his unseemly fondness for face paint and belly shirts.)

The Stud (Yul Brynner): Whether playing cowboy with his six magnificent companions or regally resplendent in the garb of a Siamese king, Yul Brynner was the original bald badass of stage and screen. It's all in the eyes; with a glare that intense, you could get away with wearing a diaper. (And if you're in chemotherapy long enough, you may eventually get a chance!)

The Megalomaniac (Lex Luthor): Sure, his single-minded obsession with besting Superman and ruling the world won't win him any popularity contests; when it comes to fashion, Lex is no villain, looking equally stylish in elegantly tailored three-piece suits and Kryptonite-powered body armor. What's his secret? He's the richest man in the world, dummy!

The Good Leader (Patrick Stewart): As Captain Jean-Luc Picard in *Star Trek: The Next Generation* and Professor Xavier in *X-Men,* Stewart set a standard for steady, compassionate authority. Fathers, managers, military officers, and members of the clergy should all consider following his example. Essential fashion accessories for this look include Starfleet insignias and psychic powers.

The Man About Town (Telly Savalas): If you've seen an episode of *Kojak* or an old Players Club International commercial, you know that Telly Savalas is one slick son of a bitch—the kind of smooth operator who'll charm your pants off while you're losing your shirt to him at blackjack. To achieve the Savalas look, match your bald head with a trench coat, sunglasses, and a lollipop. You'll look like a king of the city—now who loves ya, baby?

The Nutcase (G. Gordon Liddy): Were you ever caught committing political sabotage? Did you ever host a talk radio show that allowed you to spit bile and paranoia into the public airwaves? Did you ever guest-star on *Miami Vice*? If you said "yes" to any of these questions, congratulations: You're already following in the footsteps of

Watergate break-in artist and ultraconservative psychopath G. Gordon Liddy. Now, if you could just grow a creepy mustache, your transformation would be complete.

The Magician (Mr. Clean): Mr. Clean doesn't just keep it clean on the kitchen floors; this tile-scrubbing genie brings the same cleanliness and simplicity to his apparel. If you have the upper body definition to show it off, then bright, tight, and white may be the perfect look for you. Penny-pinchers note: Since plain T-shirts will only run you a few bucks apiece, this style won't thin out your wallet the way chemo thinned out your hair.

Guides to the Planet

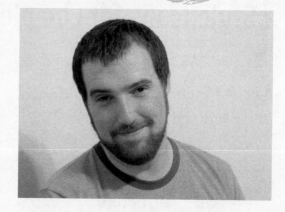

Curtis Luciani was twenty-six years of age when he learned that his left testicle, after nothing but years of peaceful cohabitation, had decided to kill him by going all Stage II cancer-y. Trained medical professionals unleashed surgical and chemical hell upon the wayward testicle, and Curtis is now in remission. He is an e-learning writer and sometime comedian in Austin, Texas.

Wigs

It's amazing how much of your self-esteem is wrapped up in your hair. In the beginning, I cried hardest when I knew I was going to "look" like a cancer patient rather than feel like one.
—ALICIA D.

Maybe it's just me, but it felt wrong to wear it. I felt like I was trying to hide what was really going on to make other people more comfortable.
—RED85

I don't mind my wig, since it actually looks better than my real hair did, but sometimes I'm just not in the mood, so I trade off between it and some pretty Russian-ish scarves.
—CAITLIN

For many cancer patients, hair loss is the worst part. If you feel like shit, some say, you can power through it as long as your appearance doesn't indicate that you're tired and foggy and cranky because of the chemicals your body is laboring to process. But make all of your hair fall out and have your appearance change accordingly, and there goes your ability to hide anything. And let's be honest: There's a certain psychological advantage to looking "normal," because in many cases it helps you to feel more normal. Some of Planet Cancer's denizens eschew wigs in favor of hats and bandannas or even baldness (see "The Wig-Off" later in the chapter); but for others, wigs are a great solution to tempering the physical (and emotional) change brought about by hair loss.

Below is a lot of useful counsel about wigs. Thanks to the fine people at Cancer and Careers (www.cancerandcareers.org) for sharing.

Before You Buy

ASK YOUR DOCTOR

Not all treatments cause hair loss, so discuss the possibility with your doctor. If there is a high probability you will lose some of your hair, get a prescription for a "cranial prosthesis" from your insurance company (most cover wigs needed for medical purposes). Also, ask how long it will take before your hair starts falling out and whether there are steps you can take to help retain your hair.

CALL YOUR HAIRSTYLIST

When you book your appointment, let the receptionist know you'll need some extra time, and ask if there is some place private you can talk. If not, request a slow time of the day. As the person who knows you, your hair and, most likely, other clients with cancer, a hairdresser can be a great resource. He or she may be able to suggest a local wig shop or even order one for you. Once you've bought the wig, your stylist can trim and style it for your face.

TAKE A SHORT CUT

Even if you have always worn your hair long, getting a short haircut is one of the biggest breaks you can give yourself during treatment. Long hair, pulled down by gravity, is more likely to fall out sooner. Short hair masks initial hair loss better and makes less of a mess when it does fall out. Just remember to keep a good-size lock of hair to use as a guide for wig shopping.

GIVE YOURSELF OPTIONS

Since wigs can be uncomfortable and troublesome, you probably won't want to wear one every day, all day. A hairpiece peeking out from under a hat or scarf can give the illusion of hair without the annoyance and bulk of a wig. Most wig stores and cancer specialty shops stock a wide variety of bangs, side pieces, ponytails, curls, and falls. Many of these are designed to be Velcro-ed into a hat.

Where to Buy

Besides asking your stylist, call the American Cancer Society or ask your doctor for recommendations on wig retailers and wig salons. Many shopping malls and department stores have a fun-wig shop at the very least, but you may want more privacy and a higher quality of service that a wig salon offers.

If you can't afford a wig, CancerCare (800-813-HOPE) and the American Cancer Society provide free wigs to those in need.

No matter where you go, make sure you're comfortable with the store and the staff. Call beforehand and make sure the store or wig salon specializes in cancer patients, offers refitting, can provide a private area for try-ons, and has a variety of choices, including hairpieces. Also, find out if you can try on the wigs and return them (many state's health regulations prohibit this).

You can purchase wigs online, but there's no way to tell what you are buying until it arrives at your door. If you do buy a wig over the Web, be sure you can return it for any reason.

Choosing a Wig

A wide range of factors will influence your choice of wigs: human hair or synthetic; short or long; custom- or machine-made; and price (which can range from $40 to more than $4,000).

Synthetic vs. Human Hair

Most women prefer synthetic hair. It's easier to maintain and less expensive. Most synthetic wigs have their style molded into them, but some can be reset. The advantage to wigs that can be styled is that you can change their look, just as with real hair. The disadvantage is that they have to be reset every time they're washed. Synthetic hair also dries faster than real hair. Well-made synthetic wigs may look real, but they never totally feel or move the way real hair does. Nor can you treat them like your own hair—they fry when exposed to heat. So no curling irons or blow dryers unless they are specifically designed for wigs. Hot rollers can be used, but only at low settings. And avoid exposing the wig to any intense heat sources such as an oven. The blast of heat will cause frizzing.

Wigs made of human hair will obviously look and feel more like your hair, but they are expensive, starting at $1,000, and far more time-consuming. You can use heated appliances on them for touch-ups, but you'll probably want to take them to a professional to be washed and styled.

Wig Construction

The way a wig is made affects how it looks just as much as, if not more than, the type of hair used. There are three types of wigs: custom, handmade, and machine-made.

- Machine-made wigs are the least expensive and most widely available. If you've ever worn a wig, this is probably the type you are familiar with. Wefts of hair are sewn together in a straight line, cut, and assembled into a wig. (When you look inside a machine-made wig, you can see the lines.) Many look realistic as long as they are not parted, pulled back, or otherwise altered.

Some women find these wigs more comfortable because the construction creates vents that allow air to circulate to the scalp.

- Handmade wigs look the most natural of the prefabricated choices because individual strands are knotted on to a skullcap rather than wefts of hair being sewn together. These wigs can be parted and styled with accessories because there is no chance the vents will be exposed. The hair also falls and moves more naturally.

- Custom wigs are almost indistinguishable from natural hair. They are usually not a viable option for cancer patients, as they are extremely expensive and generally take more than two months to complete. Make sure that you have final approval on the choice of hair and style.

Style

Some women use this as a time to experiment with a number of looks; others just want a wig that looks like their hair. Either way, a few adjustments can make your wig look as natural as possible.

- Keep in mind that a wig cannot replicate the way your hair blends into your skin. Sure, it does in movies, but that requires a great deal of time, makeup, and a team of trained professionals. For your purposes, bangs, or at least wisps of hair covering the hairline, will help your wig look more natural.

- Even if you're staying with the cut you currently have, try a slightly shorter wig. During treatment, many women lose weight and become slightly drawn. A shorter style can add fullness. Plus, short wigs have less hair to brush out at night and don't tangle as easily.

- Wigs that use wide headbands along the hairline are easy to wear and stylish, but you're locked into wearing a headband. Such models are better for occasional use or as a backup.

- Buying two wigs in different styles can make life easier than purchasing one very expensive wig. You won't have to restyle your wig every time you want to put your hair up.

Wigcessories

Besides the wig, you'll need some supplies: a head form to store the wig on, a wire wig brush, hairnets, T-pins to hold the wig in place while brushing, low-alcohol or wig hair spray, baby or wig shampoo, conditioner, and, depending on the length, hairpins and rollers. All are available at the wig shop, a beauty supply retailer, through your hairdresser, or online.

Wearing Your Wig

The wig shop or your hairdresser can demonstrate how to put your wig on properly by grasping it in the front and rolling it back over your head. Line up the points on the side of the wig in front of your ears, where a man's sideburns start.

As hair loss progresses, it may become difficult to tell where your natural hairline is. It's easy to wind up wearing a wig too low or too high on your forehead. Keep a photo that shows your natural hairline to use as a guide.

Under any type of wig, you'll need to wear a cap. These are soft, snug nylon or cotton cover-

167

ings that protect your scalp, control your hair, and keep the wig from slipping. Buy more caps than you think you will need; it's good to have extras and rotate them regularly.

Your wig may need to be refitted after you lose your hair, particularly if you had long or thick hair when you purchased it. Most wigs have adjustable straps at the back to change the size; if the wig still feels loose, take it back to the store for adjustment.

Caring for Your Wig

All wigs require a certain amount of daily care, but probably less than the time you'd spend on your own hair. For more information, Look Good . . . Feel Better (www.lookgoodfeelbetter.org) offers group and private instruction on wearing and maintaining wigs.

Daily Care

- When you take off your wig, store it on a Styrofoam, wood, or cloth-covered head form.

- Smooth out the hair with a comb.

- Pin short styles to set curls; roll or twist longer styles and secure with pins.

- Lightly spray with low-alcohol hair spray if desired and let dry.

- Cover with a hairnet.

- Store away from heat, dust, and humidity.

WASHING AND SETTING

If worn regularly, you'll want to wash and set your wig every week or two. Synthetic wigs can be washed and styled at home or taken to your hairstylist or wig shop. Human hair is more difficult to handle, so it's best left to professionals.

WASHING

- Brush wig with a wire wig brush, starting at the ends and working up to the scalp.

- Submerge wig in a bowl or sink of cool water and baby shampoo or soap for wigs. Gently swish.

- Soak for five minutes.

- Rinse in cool water.

- If desired, condition hair with a product for wigs or a conditioner with lanolin.

- Rinse again in cool water.

- Gently squeeze out water—do not twist.

- Place wig on a tall, slender object like a hair spray can so air can circulate through the wig.

- Allow to air-dry completely. Never brush a wet wig. (Only blow-dry if the manufacturer recommends it.)

- Gently brush from ends to scalp with wig brush.

SETTING

Most synthetic wigs have the style molded into the hair, so simply control and emphasize the set with hot rollers set on medium or low. (Never use curling irons or hair dryers on synthetic wigs.)

{ Big Wig Love }

by Patti Rogers

{ My wig made me feel like the fresh, salon blow-out version of me. }

It's true that it seems absurd to give two hoots about hair when you're staring an unexpected diagnosis in the face. At a time when life's priorities are so quickly reset and you find yourself with wide-eyed gratitude gulping down life's true gifts like shots of Red Bull for the soul, it seems wildly off-base to care about your hair. But nonetheless, cancer, chemo, and impending baldness are enough to make any of us seriously freak out!

At first, a modest few strands will start to drop. But as the days following your first round of chemo progress, you might find yourself paranoid that your hair is going to fall out all at once, perhaps at some unforeseen public moment, like standing in line at Starbucks. I for one feared getting the dreaded, friendly tap on the shoulder, "Excuse me, Miss, a blond squirrel just fell off your head." This would be the moment I would try to pretend to be an ordinary patron—nonchalantly kneeling down to gather up my nest of hair, cramming it in my purse like a handful of coins. All the while keeping my cool as I completed the complicated macchiato order, and never losing eye contact with my barista.

Whether you let it fall out, one painful, traumatic strand at a time, or whether you organize a girl gathering and sip champagne through a ceremonial shaving, is a personal choice. But the real question is "To Wig or Not to Wig?"

I considered all my options: the bare bald look, hats, scarves, bandannas, synthetic and human hair wigs. While all of them have their advantages, my personal head shield of choice was the human hair (h2) wig. Why? Because girl, that thing made me feel great.

My wig made me feel like the fresh, salon blow-out version of me. It took me the same amount of time to get ready for a nap as it did for a night out. I could go to a social function and people would say, "You look great! I thought you had cancer!" In this season of being poked, prodded, tested, and kicked in the ass, anything that makes you feel or look a little better is absolutely a bonus. And anything that helps you salvage even 1 percent of your personal swagger is a must-have.

At my hairdresser's urging, I took the h2 wig to him so he could cut it to look less off-the-rack (or, in this case, off the Styrofoam head). Then my lovely colorist added low lights. After decades of spending money to get my roots taken out, it was a strange and twisted irony to now pay someone to put them in. But, truth be told, this made all the difference in making the h2 wig look even more like my real hair. And even though I had imagined that I might be that girl who rocked a lot of different sassy styles and bright colored wigs (being a longtime Jennifer Garner *Alias* fan), in the end, what made me feel best was to feel as close to normal as possible.

Even though "normal" isn't a desirable, prime-time feature these days, in cancer-ville, anonymity can be quite appealing. I am not suggesting a denial of reality—cancer is what it is, after all. But it is nice to have a choice on when and where you "out" your platelet count to the Joe-Schmo universe.

A good wig helps you blend in on the sidelines of the fourth-grade basketball game, a nice alternative to being the game's halftime show. And if you're going out to meet your girlfriends for happy hour, it is reassuring to know that if people are craning to look at you, it will be because you look like a hottie, not because they are wondering what kind of cancer you have or if you are allowed to drink that wine. You can stand in line at the grocery store, pretending not to be reading tabloid headlines without receiving the empathetic head-tilt "hello" from the checker.

The wig gives you the choice, and styling the h2 wig is as easy as dropping off your dry cleaning. Any wig salon or wig-trained hairdresser will wash and blow-dry your "girl" while you do errands or go back home for a nap. (Helllooo, can you say "silver lining"?)

Of course, there are also plenty of times to go with the bandanna, scarf, or ball cap. These are absolutely preferred getups at the gym, around the house, at the pool, or on a walk in the neighborhood. *Note:* Wigs and sweat don't mix. No need to try.

There are plenty of other things to learn about the wig world that you will surely uncover on your own. But I must give you one warning: Wig shopping can

Guides to the Planet

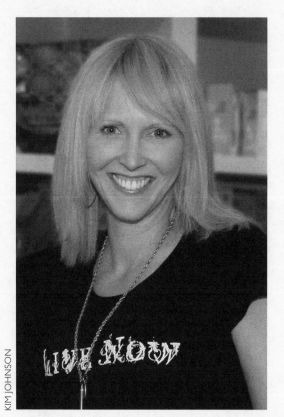

KIM JOHNSON

Patti Rogers, an Austinite since 1971, grew up as one of four girls. She has been blissfully married for fourteen years and is a proud mom of two young kids and one annoyingly large dog. On Halloween of 2008, in full Batgirl attire, she was diagnosed with Stage I breast cancer. After her lumpectomy, tests revealed the tumor was aggressive and she carried the BRCA2 gene. She did six glamorous rounds of TAC chemotherapy, followed by an oophorectomy and a double mastectomy. Eleven months later, her pathology is clear and she considers cancer to be one of life's most wonderful, imperfect gifts—giving her family more white space on the calendar, a cherished appreciation for her community and friends, and a new perspective on choosing joy each and every day. Today she pursues her yoga, writing, and whenever possible, an excuse to be Batgirl.

be a bit bizarre (maybe even a twisted cross between *Pulp Fiction* and *Steel Magnolias*). It's an experience where you will likely meet a host of memorable characters, from the aging shop owners to the passionate stylists, and of course dozens of stoic women with chiseled features, Styrofoam heads, and names like "Maria," "Stevie," "Tara," and "Savannah."

But it is worth pushing through to find the hairstyle or head shield that helps you rock your way through cancer. In a weird way, I think the wig has power. Not comic book character power and not the kind of power you'll find written up in medical journals. But a power that helps you find your normal, keep your swagger, and maybe even sport a hair-toss and a belly laugh.

Any day, any hour, any minute you can stack up feeling "good" against "not so good" is a victory in my book. The fight against cancer doesn't just happen in chemo clinics and radiation rooms. It happens in the heart. We summon our strength from wherever we can—love, laughter, prayers, and, sometimes, even the wig.

{ Leave the Wig at Home }

by Lauren Rachel Ainsworth

To many of us ladies, the prospect of losing our hair due to treatment is an issue as serious as, er, cancer. It's understandable. After chemotherapy, you go from hearing the words, "Nice 'do," to saying, "Oh, ew," as hair makes a daily appearance on your pillow—and on your shoulders, your clothes, your dinner plate, the floor, etc. That cool spring breeze becomes less enjoyable when it renders enough force to blow your bangs off. When creating a new hole in the ozone layer in an attempt to shellac it together, and all your best efforts to salvage your coif fail, you're left with a tough decision. Wear a wig, a scarf, a hat, a football helmet, anything; or risk being mistaken for an avid Trekkie.

Wigs can be alluring at first. Some are cheap, some are expensive; some real hair, some fake. The one factor that unites all wigs is their ability to offer even the slightest feeling of normalcy. They allow you to remain anonymous. Encounters with unknowing individuals remain the same. You still look decent when you really feel like shit; you look the same when you are really different.

However, the quality of this illusion can fade rather quickly. Wigs are horrendously uncomfortable. The standard woven wig makes your head itch worse than a case of poison oak that made it down to your nether regions. Newfangled adhesive hairpieces feel OK at first, but after a while your sweat loosens the adhesive, and your part slowly makes its way over to your ear. And seriously, no matter how realistic the wig or how strong the adhesive, you couldn't fool a legally blind person once your eyebrows fall out.

So, wear a hat instead. Find a couple of cool scarves at a vintage shop. Or go bald and freak some kids out. Go ahead and get a wig or two, but don't feel as if you have to wear them anywhere besides your cousin's wedding. When you have no hair, the beauty of your face is all anyone can see anyway.

Religion / Spirituality

I just haven't figured out why most people who would never directly bring up religion with a relative stranger suddenly do so when cancer or some other life-threatening ailment is involved.

—KYLE

Your take on things spiritual is about as personal as it gets, and there's nothing like a stare-down with your own mortality to provoke some thoughts about it. Some embrace religion as a powerful support that helps them find meaning in the face of a life-threatening cancer diagnosis; others go to the opposite extreme, which can result in self-imposed isolation or a more pointed spurning of religion itself.

What's important to take in about religion and spirituality—that is, any religious faith, any spirituality—is that it doesn't hurt to use this time to explore where you stand on the spirituality continuum and figure out what you're comfortable with. Whether it's to find a community beyond your close group of friends or to explain to the kindly hospital chaplain that you're happy to talk with him as long as he doesn't proselytize, getting a firmer idea about where your spiritual views stack up will help you as you navigate the Planet.

Cancer Prank

The Scalp: Slowly scratch your head. Over several seconds, scratch with increasing vigor, drawing the attention of people you don't know. When the audience is big enough, suddenly pull your wig off.

{ When I Finally Trusted in My Faith }

by Valerie Ward

One therapy that really seemed to help me relax was prayer and meditation. I had read that our subconscious mind can actually direct the healing in our body. I went on prayer walks, went to healing prayer services, and committed Bible verses on healing to memory. I visualized piranhas eating my cancer cells, roaring rivers washing all the bad stuff away, Jesus going through my body with a bright light, and angels dancing on my cancerous tissues with healing potions in their feet. I would see myself well again with no cancer. I just let the images come.

But there was still a nagging fear in the back of my mind. With everything I was throwing at my brain, was I really getting through to my subconscious? Was I really starting to believe that I could be healed? Were my prayers getting through to our Creator? Did I have enough faith?

One night near the end of my chemo treatments, I had a dream. I was sitting on a big plane getting ready for takeoff. I was sitting on the right side of the airplane in the row over the wing. As we started to take off, the plane began veering erratically to the left and right. The pilots seemed to have no control over the plane. We took off and as I looked out the window, we were skimming the tops of trees. I also saw power lines and telephone poles flying by outside my window. I thought frantically, *We're going to crash! We're going to crash!*

To my horror, the right wing hit one of the telephone poles. It was badly damaged with a big chunk missing. As I continued to stare out the window in fear, the wing slowly started to become whole again. To my shock and amazement, the missing piece of the wing grew back into place. The wing appeared as though it had never been damaged, and the plane ride became smooth. A gentle calm encased me. My tumor had, incidentally, been on the right side of my body, the same side as the damaged wing in the dream. Like that damaged wing, I was becoming whole again.

I awoke the next morning so excited about my dream that I called friends and family. From that moment on, I never doubted that I was being completely healed. The fear still pops in, especially near checkups, but I know that God hears our prayers and belief in healing is powerful.

{ Handy Ways to Hold On to Your Lack of Faith }

by Curtis Luciani

If you are ever so fortunate to be diagnosed with cancer, you will discover that it is essential to "get in touch with your spiritual side." You will discover this because every book, support group, self-help audiotape, or chatty chemotherapy nurse you turn to will tell you exactly that. And it isn't bad advice. If being "spiritual" means being in touch with the universe or having a sense of reverence—well, who's against that? And if you already find nourishment for your spiritual side in the teachings of a traditional religion, great.

However, if you don't adhere to any of the world's accredited religions, you may find that certain overeager friends or relations will have very specific ideas about exactly how poor, suffering you should get in touch with your spiritual side. These attempts to prepare your soul for its final reward will invariably be well intentioned, but they'll drain precious mental energy better used to steel yourself for the next chemo or radiation treatment.

Here, then, are a few simple tips for the cancerous atheist/agnostic. These will help you deflect well-meaning proselytes and make it through your cancer journey with your skepticism intact.

- **Adopt a "zany" religion as cover.** Like your freshman year of college, your cancer experience is a sacred time when you cannot be judged for temporarily dallying with any ideology you please. Take advantage of this; if your mother is begging you to return to regular churchgoing, ward her off by taking up Scientology or worship of the ancient Norse pantheon. When you are in remission, you can casually discard your new "faith" without consequence.

- **Have a dark night of the soul.** Even your most devout friends won't step to you if you pretend that getting cancer has locked you in an epic, Job-like struggle with the higher power. It's easy: Stare darkly out a window for about an hour, then turn your gaze to the heavens, shake a fist defiantly, and scream, "Why?" (For more tips on dark nights of the soul, consult the films of Ingmar Bergman.)

- **Go science crazy!** Obtain exhaustive technical knowledge of your disease. Spout statistics at the drop of a hat. Run down all the steps you are taking to get better, and detail the impact of each of them on a cellular level. When your religious friends see that you've gone 100 percent empirical, they'll pack up their power of prayer and leave you be.

{ **The Religion Diner** }

by Carrie Morse

After I started treatment, I started dining a la carte at the "Religion Diner." Hmmm, let's see. Prayer lists? Sure. Add my name to them all. Figured I could use as many prayers as possible. Tibetan prayer flags? Hell yeah! I'll hang those in my apartment in a place where they'll catch a breeze and move. In fact, they're still up. Not taking them down anytime soon! Light a candle? Sure, I love candles. Light a hundred of them. Pray to the saints? Bring it. I love the saints.

A good friend of my mom's sent me a St. Peregrine medal. He's the patron saint of those with cancer. I'm not Catholic, but I wore that medal on a bracelet every day from the time I received it until my onc said I was in remission. Once in a while I wear it again just for good measure. I met with and continue to meet with the amazing minister at my parents' Methodist church in Birmingham, Michigan. He's been a tremendous source of support and guidance. He also gave me some great pointers for dealing with people who told me that everything would be fine, "if you just believe."

I basically looked over the menu and picked what worked for me. And one year post-treatment, I still haven't made any firm decisions. I'm still looking over the menu.

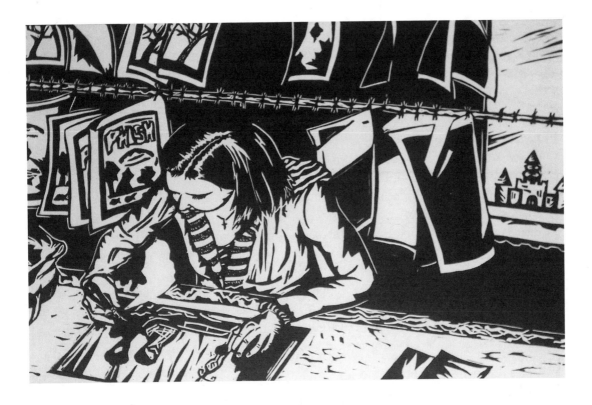

The Art of Cancer

During treatment (and after), you'll notice that time will likely become more important to you. Or perhaps not more important, but more noticeable. First, time is dictated by your treatment schedule, like a countdown: *Two weeks until chemo. Tomorrow, and the day after, the day after that, and then for the rest of the month, I have radiation at 11:30.* Or: *When the hell are they going to call with my CBC results?* Each day—each milestone—passes, and you feel it.

It becomes important to many people to create a context for this passage of time. Making playlists for different moods, whether you're pissed at being lethargic, happy to be done with another chemo session, or somewhere in between, is one example. Or writing in a journal, repainting your room graffiti-style, or making a documentary at the hospital featuring your docs and nurses and family and a bunch of anonymous people whose butts stick out of their hospital gowns. It all helps.

Music, painting, talking into a digital voice recorder, carrying a camera around—any creative outlet helps you cope with cancer and your treatment. You might not even know that as you draw a pencil sketch of your doctor, this helps you create a context within which you're processing what's happening to you on your own terms. Picasso said, "Art washes away from the soul the dust of everyday life." And really, for you in the here and now, what's more important than that?

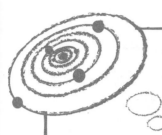

Dispatches
from the Planet

I wanted a way to give something back. Humor was one of the things that I used to help myself deal with those bad chemo days. It was how I coped with the daily issues of treatment. Humor was a distraction. If I sat and thought about how bad the chemo was going to make me feel, I'd almost start to get sick. I'd make jokes, like "Hmmm, what do I want to throw up for lunch tomorrow!" Laughter had a way of making it all good for a while. I knew that if I could spread that humor around, I could make people smile, maybe even share a laugh with someone. And for that moment that they're laughing, they're not thinking of cancer. It's sort of like being cancer-free for an instant!

I came up with the idea that T-shirts were the way to go. I could deliver the T-shirts, and the T-shirts would deliver the message. Being a software developer by trade, I knew I could build the Web site, which would then open it up to the world.

The site's primary goal is to put a smile on the faces of those in the fight against cancer. Humor is good medicine. A simple T-shirt that spoofs cancer can make the person wearing the T-shirt feel good, brighten a room when everyone sees it, and start a conversation between those who know cancer all too well. Proceeds from got-Cancer.org are used to support various cancer charities. So far, that list includes Planet Cancer, Heavenly Hats, and Cancer Sucks, all grassroots cancer nonprofits. gotCancer.org also sponsors teams and individuals in fund-raising events such as Race for the Cure and Relay for Life.

—Larry Mull

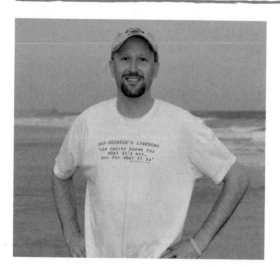

Guides
to the Planet

Larry Mull was diagnosed at age thirty-five with Stage II large cell, aggressive non-Hodgkin's lymphoma. The good doctors figured that out after they sliced out about seven centimeters of his small intestine. Next came six rounds of the chemo cocktail, R-CHOP. After that, he writes, "They decided to fry up anything that

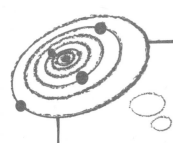

Dispatches from the Planet

My husband, Dale, and I are performers down here at the Jersey shore. We have our very own rock band, Goodbie Amy. He's the guitar player, and I am the singer. Now don't get too excited, because we are only one of those "local cover bands." Hey, it's money! Have you ever stopped to think about how doing what you love to do helps you forget your troubles? Well, after I was diagnosed with cancer, I followed my doctors' orders, but unless I had drains hanging from my body and/or gaping wounds, I was on that stage singing and performing and doing what I love to do! It truly helped me in my healing.

—*Amy L. Paradise*

Although I wanted to find my own identity, I just couldn't declare my independence as a dependent cancer patient. And although there were positive aspects to being treated in a children's hospital, the downside was being a young adult but being treated like a child. So most of my days were spent trying to score some piece of age-appropriateness in a sea of Disney murals and visiting clowns.

To manage, I mostly did crafts and played video games. I also shunned "candy stripers" and anyone else who wanted to label me with juvenile treatment. My escape came between treatments when I could go home to eat fudge ice cream and paint my nails blue with cheap, sticky nail polish.

But my true solace came on the nights when I couldn't fall asleep. It was then that I would tiptoe downstairs to watch *Cartoon Sushi*, a show of twisted and artistic animated shorts. I would laugh and snicker at the rudimentary characters and crass plotlines that mocked popular cartoon culture. My fun didn't stop there, because next *120 Minutes* would come on. I would stare in wonderment at the Buffalo Daughter, Cibo Matto, and Radiohead music videos. They were unlike anything I had ever seen before, and they made me realize that I could one day be that creative.

Those sleepless nights have affected everything in my life from the high school I attended to my majors in college. They made me dream, and they kept my hopes up during treatment.

—*Cambrey Thomas*

was left with seventeen doses of external beam radiation therapy." Six years later, his oncologist has told him that he doesn't want to see him anymore. The radiation specialists won't even let him take rides through the CT scanner anymore. He counts himself lucky to be a successful statistic, able to spend time with his girls: his wife, Chris, and daughter, Lauren.

What it's really like to . . .
Cut a Cancer-Themed Rap Album

by Jesse Hershkowitz, aka Urbalist

This is how hip-hop saved my life. The album *Cancerous Flow: Lyrical Journal* is a rap album that I wrote, produced, and recorded while undergoing intense chemotherapy to beat non-Hodgkin's lymphoma. Each song on the album is a look into the mind of a cancer patient in the midst of the battle. The creative process of making the album saved my life and made me able to mentally deal with chemo treatment.

I first came up with the idea for the album after my initial diagnosis. I went to my bedroom and locked the door and didn't come out for two days. I realized I could not just sit passively through six months of treatment. I desperately needed an outlet and a way to occupy myself. I had been a rapper, songwriter, and producer for ten years, and hip-hop music was always how I expressed myself. I played with different ideas on how to channel the emotions I was and would be feeling in the upcoming months.

Once I had decided to do the album, I began coming up with song concepts and writing lyrics. I completed all the writing for the songs first. I had to spend a total of thirty-six days inpatient, so I was unable to record then, but when I was home, I recorded all the songs in a studio that I set up in a spare bedroom in my parents' house.

I was in the vocal booth with my chemo backpack laying down lyrics and recording songs at every available moment. I had a friend of mine from Rhode Island, Edgar "Vertigo" Cruz, mix down the songs and add some extra instruments to the beats. By the time my treatment was done, I had finished the album.

> I was in the vocal booth with my chemo backpack laying down lyrics and recording songs at every available moment.

Since putting out *Cancerous Flow: Lyrical Journal,* my entire musical direction and goals have changed. We donate copies of the album to Memorial Sloan-Kettering Cancer Center, where I was treated, and they give them out to the adolescents and young adults. I've performed songs from the album at a number of American Cancer Society Relay for Life events in New Jersey and am featured on Vol. 2 of the *I'm Too Young for This Benefit* compilation CD.

From the song "The First Five Days," from *Cancerous Flow: Lyrical Journal:*

Now I could give up all hope,
but nope, not me,
I've been to places so dangerous
that most cops flee.
So you see, I'm not afraid and I ain't choosin'
despair,
Not even if I'm nauseous all day and losing
my hair.

Guides to the Planet

Jesse Hershkowitz has been writing and producing both his own and others' music since he was fifteen years old. He officially became a cancer survivor in February 2007, when he finished his last chemotherapy treatment. Learn more about Jesse on YouTube, where you can see a documentary film about him called *Back to Life.*

Cancerous Flow: Lyrical Journal is for sale on Jesse's MySpace page (www.myspace.com/urbriskitallrep); sales benefit Memorial Sloan-Kettering Cancer Center, where he received treatment.

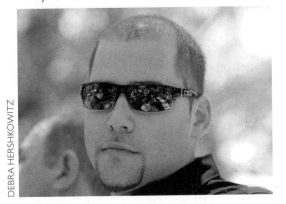

DEBRA HERSHKOWITZ

{ Journal Writing }

by Jen Slaski

OK, let's get something out of the way up front: Journal writing is not writing as you may know (and fear!) it. For many, the word "writing" conjures up the trappings of a graded English composition—proper spelling and grammar, fluid cadence and sentence structure, all the formalities that suggest it's for others' consumption and judgment. The good news? Journal writing is not about pomp and circumstance that's on display. It is for one person alone: you. And all it requires is for you to show up, pen in hand, and be willing to put on paper what's swirling around in your head and heart. To be willing to acknowledge and honor what's happening in your life. And in the process, get to the heart of you and get on to the business of healing so that you can make the most of today.

While an incredibly useful daily practice in even the most ordinary of times, journal writing can be an especially helpful tool in getting through the blindsiding chapters of life that deliver anything but what we had planned. Coming to terms with life when it's not what we envisioned is traumatic. A heartbreaking disappointment, an unexpected diagnosis, the death of a loved one. All of these events involve the trauma wreaked by loss—whether it's loss of what we believed reality to be, the vision of what our future would be, or even just the control we fooled ourselves into thinking we had in those matters. And these realizations of loss are accompanied by a deluge of new and overwhelming emotions that we may not feel quite prepared—even equipped—to deal with.

Journal writing is a way of acknowledging and dealing (sometimes coping!) with these emotions. To rant, rave, and rage. To quietly lament and feel sad or even gutted. To encourage ourselves to see the light of possibility. To do whatever you feel you must to be authentic about what has happened, how you feel about it, where you are today, and where you want to go tomorrow. We can try to push these thoughts and feelings to the fringe and continue on our merry way as though nothing has changed. But the mind-body-spirit connection has a tricky way of ensuring that they will always catch up with us. If ignored, they'll find a way to get noticed, manifesting in everything from sleeplessness, anxiety, and depression to a weakened immune system that resists regeneration and recovery.

Dr. James Pennebaker, Ph.D., professor and chair of the Department of Psychiatry at the University of Texas in Austin and author of *Writing to Heal: A Guided Journal for Recovering from Trauma & Emotional Upheaval,* has conducted numerous research studies on how journal writing has a positive impact on health and healing—both from an emotional and a physical perspective. His findings have shown everything from how journal writing is positively correlated with faster healing of war vets' wounds to fewer clinic visits for homesick or heartbroken college students. While there are plenty of scientific left-brain/right-brain theories, much of it boils down to the mind-body-spirit connection. Following the steps below can help you get started on exploring how journal writing can help you tap into that connection and help you along your current path.

How to Get Started Writing a Journal

1. GET A JOURNAL.

A journal is simply a blank book that you know is private. It can have lines or no lines, be a leather-bound masterpiece or an old-school composition notebook. The key is that it is yours and that you feel secure that whatever you write will be for your eyes only (unless you choose to share it with someone else).

2. GET A FREE-FLOWING PEN.

Get a pen that allows you to write easily and to keep up with your train of thought. One that allows you to fly across the page, capture the stream-of-consciousness voice in your head, and not worry about what your handwriting looks like. Some experts advise writing in green ink because it evokes creativity and allows us to be less inhibited in our writing. But whether black, blue, green, or orange, fancy fountain pen or old-school Bic, just choose whatever works.

3. FIND FIVE MINUTES BY YOURSELF.

Start writing in your journal as if you were beginning to train for a running race. Just five minutes to begin with. Then work your way up to ten minutes, then fifteen. Before you know it, it will take on a life of its own, and you'll find the right amount of time you need to get out of it what you must. You'll know you've struck the right balance when you close your journal feeling a sense of relief and clarity.

As for when you write in your journal, some experts say morning is the best time to write because it's when your ego (that typically scoffs at things like writing in a journal!) is most relaxed after a night of sleep. But really, anytime is better than not at all, so do it in the morning in your kitchen, at the coffee shop in the afternoon, on your back porch as the sun goes down, or at night as you're turning in. Do it wherever. The important thing is to do it at a time and in a place where no one will interrupt you or ask you to share what you are doing. Because remember, writing in a journal is all about you being able to share freely with no one other than you.

4. READY, SET . . . WRITE!

Write whatever comes to you at that moment. What's most on your mind, bothering you, what you dreamed about that you remember, what happened earlier this week that has been gnawing at you . . . whatever's struck you and has been lingering. Even if you just start out with "Today I am feeling . . . ," you'll be amazed at what can come from that simple starting point if you don't try to do anything but finish that thought authentically.

Some people get paralyzed by this "openness" and prefer a bit more structure, which is natural. In this case, writing prompts help. Go through this list and see which prompt speaks to you or go through the list one at a time. When you're done, go through the prompts again! Over time, you will naturally come up with your own.

JOURNAL PROMPTS:

- Today, I'd like to . . .

- Something that's been on my mind is . . .

- When I was little, I always thought . . .

- My biggest challenge is . . .

- I'm so sick and tired of . . .

- I'm grateful for . . .

- Something that's surprised me . . .

- I wish that . . .

- What I've noticed recently is . . .

- If I could, I would . . .

- The single most important thing now is . . .

Also feel free to write to whomever you feel comfortable with. Some people find comfort in using their journal as a place where they just capture their own thoughts and musings, as though writing in the first person ("I am, I feel . . . "). Others prefer to direct their thoughts toward someone/something else—be that a trusted friend ("Dear Diary") or a spiritual figure (God, the Universe, etc.).

The most critical take-home point is that, as long as you are writing in your journal, there is no "right" or "wrong" topic, tone, style, form, or fashion. It is simply about whatever feels right and comfortable for you. Revel in that freedom.

5. . . . & WRITE SOME MORE!

If your first few journal-writing endeavors feel a bit awkward and less fruitful than you'd hoped or expected, fret not! Studies performed by Dr. Pennebaker have shown that it requires an average of four sessions before the benefits of journal writing can be materially experienced. This is largely because it is a new activity for so many and, as

> The most critical take-home point is that, as long as you are writing in your journal, there is no "right" or "wrong" topic.

with all new things, it may take a few tries to get into the flow and feel comfortable.

But that's not to say that you should stop at four! As with all good habits, the more you do them, the more they become part of a lifestyle with the potential to impact your life meaningfully. Developing your own style, approach, and comfort level may take a bit of time, but the more you do it the more effective it will be. Eventually, writing in your journal can even begin to feel like spending time with an old friend—one that listens and provides valuable support and insight, often at times when you didn't even ask or expect to find it.

So—there you have it: all that you need to get started on your journal writing journey! Journal writing may not be for everyone, but it's certainly worth a try, especially for anyone who's curious to explore how tapping into what's happening inside of us can help us tap into the possibility that awaits us outside in the form of today.

Good luck!

Complementary and Alternative Medicine (CAM)

Acupuncture totally helps me bounce back from chemo and does wonders for neuropathy. Oh—not sure if this counts but, probiotics: major help for those of us with GI/butt issues. Oh! One more: bourbon.

—Winediva

First, let's clarify exactly what we're talking about: CAM is defined as any medical system, practice, or product that is not considered part of conventional medicine—"conventional" meaning medicine as practiced by an M.D. (medical doctor), a D.O. (doctor of osteopathy), and their allied health professionals, such as physical therapists, psychologists, and registered nurses.

For many young adults, a lot of what mainstream medicine views as woo-woo is already mainstream: yoga, acupuncture, massage, meditation, supplements, juicing, chiropractic, and raw foods, to name a few. But when you're fighting cancer, the impact of any of these treatments or products can be magnified, for better *or* for worse. Add that there are some real scumbags out there who prey on the wallets of people in desperate health circumstances, and it's not surprising that the world of CAM can be murky and unclear.

It's important, first of all, to go in with eyes wide open. Do your research into the validity of claims made by various CAM practitioners that interest you. The phrase "too good to be true" is one to remember here. (Check out the National Center for Complementary and Alternative Medicine at http://nccam.nih.gov. This National Institutes of Health agency conducts research on CAM, trains CAM researchers, and disseminates their findings to the medical community and general public. It's a crackpot-free zone.) Second, always inform your health-care team about CAM treatments you're considering. While all doctors might not be open to CAM, your doctor might surprise you. The best docs will work with you to make sure that what you're doing, at the very least, won't hurt you, and they can also help by ordering tests and scans as objective monitors of what's going on inside your body.

Five Categories of Cam

1. **Mind-body medicine** is based on the belief that the mind can affect the body. Examples of mind-body medicine are meditation, hypnosis, yoga, biofeedback, and imagery. Other examples include any creative outlet that you enjoy, from keeping a journal to drawing, making music to dancing in front of a mirror.

Biofeedback is sometimes used for pain management or to help manage side effects. By training with various specialized machines, you learn to control certain involuntary body functions you normally wouldn't be aware of (e.g., heart rate, temperature).

Practitioners of *imagery* or visualization picture certain scenes or experiences to promote relaxation and healing. A common visualization is imagining oneself in a relaxing place, such as walking on a beach or floating in a lake. More cancer-specific visualizations might be imagining radiation as a beam of white light entering your tumor, slowly dissolving it into nothing.

A study in the December 2004 issue of the *Journal of Clinical Oncology* reported that 88 percent of 102 people with cancer who were enrolled in Phase I clinical trials at the Mayo Comprehensive Cancer Center had used at least one CAM therapy. Of those, 93 percent had used supplements (such as vitamins or minerals), 53 percent had used non-supplement forms of CAM (such as prayer/spiritual practices or chiropractic care), and almost 47 percent had used both.

2. **Biologically based practices** use natural products—vitamins, herbs, and diets tailored to your ingestion of things untainted by any chemicals—to battle cancer.

3. **Manipulative and body-based practices** work directly on the body with hands and/or other tools. Manipulative and body-based practices include massage, chiropractic care, and reflexology (the use of pressure points in the hands and feet to affect other parts of the body).

4. **Energy medicine** operates under the belief that the body has energy fields and that therapists can manipulate these fields to attain healing and wellness. Some examples:

- Tai Chi incorporates slow movements while patients focus on breathing and concentration.

- Reiki's practitioners balance energy either from a distance or by placing hands on or near the patient.

- Practitioners of therapeutic touch move their hands over the energy fields of the patient's body.

5. **Whole medical systems** incorporate healing systems from different cultures around the world:

- Ayurvedic medicine, from India, stresses balance among body, mind, and spirit.

- Chinese medicine believes that a body's good health stems from a balance of two forces called yin and yang. Acupuncture is a common practice in Chinese medicine that involves stimulating specific points on the body with needles to promote health or to lessen disease symptoms and treatment side effects.

- Homeopathy uses very small, diluted doses of substances that are supposed to bring about symptoms similar to the disease in hopes of triggering the body to heal itself.

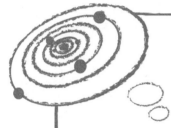

Dispatches
from the Planet

When my dad found out I had cancer, he took me to this lady, and let me tell you what an experience it was. First of all, I tried not laughing the whole entire time. She put rocks on my body and was trying to "lift" the cancer out of my body and "shoo" it away. She was saying funny things and kept making these arm movements as if she was grabbing the cancer out from my body and throwing it in the trash can. Needless to say, before we could even walk halfway out the door, I looked at my dad and said, "Thanks, but, uh … never again."

—*Princess Missy*

I did healing touch. I was diagnosed with Stage III Hodgkin's lymphoma last fall and like most, lost all my energy through chemo. Healing touch really helped me gain more energy, find my center, and even lessen the nausea. I did healing touch therapies about once a week. I loved it. I haven't done it as much since I finished treatment, but would go back in a heartbeat!

—*Trish*

Getting Help for Your Head

Once I got past the idea that talking to a professional might indicate I wasn't just cancer-ridden but crazy, too, I actually liked having the chance to vent without anyone spitting back the "Oh, I'm sure you'll be fine" platitudes. The doctors boss you around too much, and your friends and family tiptoe around you—this was right in the middle. For an hour a week, I was actually tying up all the loose ends that at times made me feel helpless.

—CC

There's no shame in going to see a professional to talk about what you're going through (or what you went through). Period. (You've been spending enough time under the care of medical professionals, we know; but this is different!) All psychological miracles aside, sometimes it helps just to discuss your mind-set with someone outside your usual group, someone who won't judge what you're saying.

In the interests of cost-effectiveness, start with the social workers at your hospital, who are trained to provide this kind of service. They will be psyched—they spend way more time than they want to dealing with insurance companies and not nearly enough time actually helping people like you cope with what you're going through.

If you'd rather go outside of your treating medical institution, insurance will often pay for your sessions with a mental health professional: a psychologist or a psychiatrist. (The difference is that a psychiatrist can write prescriptions for drugs; psychologists generally cannot.)

What's the worst thing that can happen? You don't like the first person you talk with and you switch. Then you switch again. And again. Look for a good fit—often it'll take several prospects before you find someone you're comfortable with. If you don't like any of them, don't go anymore. The bottom line is that if you feel as if you should talk with someone, do it. Hey, Tony Soprano did.

The Players

The list below outlines the roles that various professionals should play and will help you figure out who can help with the emotional and psychological aspects of cancer. That said, each person may vary in effectiveness. If you try a couple but are still in need of assistance, ask your medical team for advice or reach out to others on My Planet to see where they went.

PSYCHOLOGIST

A psychologist should be part of your medical team. Psychologists in oncology have expertise in dealing with many of cancer's effects, including depression, anxiety, insomnia, and pain. They are not just someone to talk to, but they can actually teach you techniques that you can use at home or wherever you need them for relaxation, concentration, and coping in general. The psychologist not only sees patients but should also be available to see everyone else in your family who is impacted by cancer.

Here's the rub: This service is not always covered by insurance. Check with your insurance provider before seeking services, which should be coded as a medical portion of treatment.

NEUROPSYCHOLOGIST

After some treatments, especially for brain tumors, there can be a ton of subtle and not-so-subtle changes in the way you think, organize, or memorize. These changes will impact school, work, and overall day-to-day stuff. A neuropsychologist does testing that will show you what challenges you have as well as practical ways to deal with them. Ideally you'll have some testing done when you start treatment, so you know where you were before surgery and/or treatment and can better gauge the impact. Not all treatment centers have a neuropsychologist, but your nurse practitioner or social worker should be able to recommend one. If you have or had a brain tumor, ask the person if he or she has experience in dealing with this diagnosis, as familiarity is a definite plus.

PSYCHIATRIST

Everyone deals with cancer and its effects differently, and sometimes assistance is required that includes more drugs, preferably the legal kind. These are the guys who can prescribe drugs for all of the psychological and emotional stuff, difficulties in clear thinking, and sleeping problems and anxieties you may experience as a result of cancer and its treatment. One area people really forget to deal with, don't have time to think about, or simply don't give themselves permission to talk about, is grief. Psychiatrists, psychologists, and social workers can all help you with this—their methods are just different. You have to figure out what works best for you.

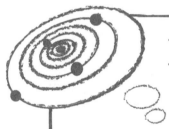

Dispatches from the Planet

In my experience psychiatrists generally won't talk to you much except for the initial consultation/diagnosis visit. After that it's just ten- or fifteen-minute checkup visits to adjust meds. Psychologists, on the other hand, are great because they can offer an unbiased opinion on what's going on, while also being able to maybe help you see another side of things you may have not noticed. It's nice to be able to have someone to talk to that's totally confidential and you don't have to worry about hurting their feelings, etc.

—MufasaProphet

I would recommend going to a psychologist. I didn't go when I was in treatment or even in the months/years following treatment. But not too long ago, I went to an acupuncturist who also happened to be a psychologist . . . and I have to say, I loved it! It felt like such a relief to be able to talk to someone with an unbiased point of view. It gave me a lot of perspective about what was going on in my life. I wished that I had gone during the years of and following my treatment.

—LauraB

One area people really forget
to deal with, don't have time to
think about, or simply don't give
themselves permission to talk
about, is grief.

What fun is the life you're
struggling to save if you don't
enjoy it even as you fight?

If this were a movie script, here we would cut to a shot of you on a Saturday night, curled up on the couch in your jammies between Mom and Dad, reaching for popcorn.

Chapter Six

People

I know now that people are basically good and want to help others. I couldn't believe how many people wanted to do whatever they could for us. Even people who didn't know us or were just acquaintances before.

—ALICIA D.

Whether you're an introvert, a family stalwart, or you party like Keith Richards, cancer will probably impact the way you interact with everyone. It will affect your family life and your social life, and will leave its fingerprints on everything in between. It can change your social desires and needs, and likely your hair (there's no medical proof of the relationship between the latter consequence and the former one). It can even change your relationship with your kids, siblings, and parents. (If this were a movie script, here we would cut to a shot of you on a Saturday night, curled up on the couch in your jammies between Mom and Dad, reaching for popcorn.)

There's no pat formula for dealing with people. The best thing to do is handle each person and situation individually and patiently—depending, of course, on your mood, energy level, and the amount of steroids in your system. (A little prednisone enters the room, and all bets are off. See 'Roid Rage in chapter 4.)

Tailoring your time with different people to your own preferences and moods—while being extra careful to allow yourself "me" time—can help you navigate all phases of your cancer experience. Be the arbiter of your own time and be unrelenting. People will understand. And if they don't, hey, you've got cancer.

If you're one of those people in the orbit of a young adult patient, there's a lot for you to learn, too. From what not to say to a young adult cancer patient, to what he or she most wants and needs, to how to take care of your friend/spouse/partner while not abandoning your own needs—it's all addressed in this chapter.

Family

I couldn't believe when, early on in my treatment, I came home—I'd moved back in with my parents—and my dad up and says, "This is so hard on me. Have you thought about that?"

—SALLYMAC

I always knew I had good parents, but I learned that in fact I have great parents. For me, nothing was harder than to watch my parents. They had the cancer as much as I did and wished they could take my place.

—HALEY MELLERT

> Be the arbiter of your own time and be unrelenting. People will understand. And if they don't, hey, you've got cancer.

There are several primary areas to keep in mind when it comes to cancer and its impact on families. While these areas are applicable to any family relationship, they become particularly important when the young adult parent has cancer.

Communication

Suffice it to say that you cannot *over*communicate when it comes to cancer and families. This is especially true when it comes to parents who have a desire to protect and shelter their children, especially younger ones, from bad news. While this impulse is admirable, it is also somewhat misguided. The reality is that kids are perceptive. Even as infants, children sense nonverbal cues when something in their environment changes, from the feeling of a port in their mother's chest to the extra people in the house to the subtle smell of chemotherapy. Big problems arise in families when information is kept under wraps and children are left to make up their own ideas about what's going on.

On the other end of the spectrum, young adults also often feel the necessity to protect their parents or siblings from their own fear, pain, or anxiety. Putting on a brave face might work for a while, but it will require an enormous amount of energy—which you probably don't have—to sustain. And then you lose an incredible opportunity to let them support you when you really need it.

Communicate with family members in honest, simple (and, for kids, age-appropriate) ways about what's going on, and they will be able to face the experience and deal with it instead of internalizing it and making up their own incredibly terrifying boogeymen. Which we all do, kids or otherwise.

{ Tips on Talking to Children about Cancer }

by Melissa Hicks, MS, CCLS, LPC, RPT
and Farya Phillips, MA, CCLS

Children are impacted by the diagnosis of a parent's serious illness in many ways, but frequently, their emotional needs and concerns can go unaddressed during times of crisis. Most children want to handle crisis in a positive way and have the potential to cope and grow through this difficult time. The following suggestions may help children to cope with an illness in the family:

- Honesty is the most important tool. Provide honest, accurate information at the child's developmental level related to the illness and its treatment.

- Use the name of the disease. Many children will hear it somewhere. If the diagnosis is explained by family members, it can help children to feel included and maintains the trust in the relationship.

- Keep children informed about your current medical status as you know it.

- Let children know that, although it is a serious disease, it does not necessarily mean the person will die from it.

- Let children know what you are doing to help treat the illness and what the side effects are. Explain changes related to energy level and mood.

- If possible, allow children the choice to go to the clinic or make hospital visits and make sure they are well prepared for what to expect.

- Be sure children understand that they did not cause the illness in any way and that it is not contagious (if this is true).

- Encourage children to ask questions. Older children may even want to ask questions of medical staff.

- Help children to know that it is OK to express their feelings and that you are willing to talk about anything they would like to discuss.

- Encourage the expression of feelings. Help children find acceptable ways to express anger.

- Allow yourself to express your emotions in front of your children. Doing so supports the idea that it is all right to feel different ways.

- Allow for alternative support people for children to talk to. They may be afraid to tell the person with the illness something for fear it may upset them.

- Keep routines as normal as possible. This predictability allows for a sense of security during an uncertain time. Explain any necessary changes in routines.

- Let children know it is OK to still have fun and do normal activities even though your family is coping with an illness.

- Reassure children that they will be cared for no matter what happens.

- Allow children to find ways to help and be included in new family routines related to the illness experience. However, be careful not to put too much additional responsibility on children.

- Watch for changes in behavior such as mood, eating, and sleeping patterns, etc.

- Inform schools about what is going on in the family, as it may impact your children's school performance.

- Be prepared to discuss difficult topics such as death.

- If possible, allow your children to interact with other children who may be facing similar life experiences. It helps them to know they are not alone.

These tips were generously provided by the amazing social workers at Wonders and Worries, a great organization that works with families and, particularly, children whose parents have cancer. Find out more at www.wondersandworries.org.

Consistency

A cancer diagnosis brings a certain loss of control—OK, a *serious* loss of control—and a sense of the world turning upside down. Kids in particular crave stability and routine, and when the family world is upended, it's worth identifying and committing to certain things that children can count on, which may help reduce stress and reground their worlds. For example: knowing that they will have a closetful of clean clothes every Monday, that they go to church with Grandma on Sundays, or that

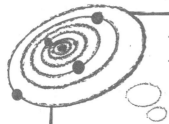

Dispatches from the Planet

My mother had to clean and organize my apartment, and I could not provide that much help. She also had to buy groceries. It is a humbling experience when your mother goes into your cabinets to organize your things, and she organizes your assortment of flavored condoms. She didn't say anything. She just did it.

Now, my brother, he decided to be politically correct and ask if I wanted to remove anything from my office before he and my mom started cleaning it. I told him no, because the only thing that had ever been inappropriate was my toy cat-of-nine-tails, and he had taken that home with him as a backscratcher the last time he visited me. (Is that the most hillbilly thing you have ever heard of? He used it as a backscratcher!)

Anyway, my mother got up and left the room. She gets embarrassed over something I don't even own anymore. I don't get it.

—*Cara Mia Massey*

Being back home is sometimes easy and sometimes hard. I deal pretty well with it, I think. But with everything going on, sometimes I freak out on my parents, which isn't fair to them. Plus it's usually unnecessary, so I feel like crap about it. I mean, they're doing so much for me—it's hard to tell them that you're an adult that needs a certain amount of space while they're doing so much for you, because you feel like an ingrate.

—*warren*

I'm a thirtysomething, independent, single guy. My parents were still overbearing, and I found that you gotta lay down the rules. Let them know you appreciate their help and you understand their concern. If they love you that much, tell them you'll keep them informed of everything. If they still persist, tell them you will formally ask the doctors to invoke HIPAA on them. Your medical team will comply. I don't suggest doing this unless you feel knowledgeable about your condition. Close personal communication with your medical team is essential.

—*cirezevlag*

they know in advance who is going to pick them up at school every day.

Boundaries

During young adulthood, you are in the process of establishing your own independent identity. How far along you are in that process depends mainly on where you are on life's continuum: from going off to college to getting married to having your own kids to taking care of your aging parents. Cancer throws a giant wrench into this process, often tossing you back into a very dependent state (for example: moving back home with your parents, being subject to the dictates of your medical team, or relying on family members for daily assistance).

These circumstances can blur the lines, but remember that just because your situation dictates physical dependence, it doesn't mean that you have to give up the hard-won emotional independence of your young adulthood. Be willing to draw a line and set boundaries, to say, "Mom/Dad/Big Brother—these are my deci-sions to make. I love you and I welcome your input and support, but I'm in charge here." You may be surprised at what a turning point it can be in your family relationships.

Self-care

The old oxygen-mask theory holds true here: Put your mask on before putting it on the child sitting with you. You can't take care of anyone else if you haven't first taken care of yourself. Whether you are the patient or a support member, if you are running on fumes, you will not be able to bring your A-game to the practical or emotional support of your family members.

While each family dynamic is unique, how hard or easy the whole experience is frequently depends on where you are in your own life—how comfortable you are taking control of your environment, asking for what you want, promoting honest communication, and setting boundaries with the people who are closest to you and have known you longer than anyone.

What it's really like to . . .
Experience Cancer with Your Twenty-Six-Year-Old Sister

by Christopher Schultz

It was the first news I'd ever heard after being told to sit down. It was winter. I was in college, a junior. I'd just come into my room after a week of midterms, and the phone rang. My sister. *How did your paper turn out?* OK. Some other stuff, small talk. When she told me that I should sit, I didn't know what to think. Were my parents splitting up? No way. Besides, they'd tell me that themselves. Did something really good happen? Had she finally gotten a kick-ass job after bartending and backpacking her way around the world? Met the right guy? I didn't think that there was anything that bad that she could possibly say.

She started retracing the past few months. *Remember when I came to visit for Parents' Weekend, and my ankle was hurting? We were dancing at that concert, and I had to kind of limp? And I came home and the doctors kept telling me that the pain was just a stone bruise from soccer, but I still couldn't even sleep?*

She went on, and I knew then. I knew it was coming, and my mind raced forward. No way. Not her. Jesus! All my life I'd heard people describe her as an angel. A friend whispered it to me when she visited me at school. She's like an angel, he said. This shit doesn't happen to angels. I hadn't sat down when she told me to—does anyone? You need to be on your feet, to run if you have to; who knows where, but that's what you feel—but I sat down then.

The word "malignant" came through, rammed its onomatopoetic leer right into my face, choked me a little. But there was something behind it—the tone that carried it, her voice, imparting the word its due weight but not giving it anything more, as a policeman might discuss a miscreant child with his parents: Ma'am, we've got a little *problem*. It brought me back, that tone. It was her, after all—my sister. She'd beat the shit out of this thing. How did I know? That voice, the first hint of a strength that I—and, I came to realize, she—never knew she had.

We went wig shopping when I was first home. She'd just gotten her hair cut above her shoulders—this way, the chemotherapy wouldn't bring about a change so drastic when her hair began to disappear. We talked about how strange it was for insurance to pay for a wig, in full, when they were so ornery about every other possible payment. We had lots of fun in the store, trying on different styles—the platinum Zsa Zsa, the impossibly spherical Supremes, the bright red Annie, the Princess Leia like a helmet. When we got to ones that approximated her hair, reminding us of why we really were there, we veered toward the practical and learned that human-hair wigs are less durable than synthetic—as if this were a surprise. We looked at before-and-after photos of chemotherapy patients whose hair had gone from straight blond to curly red, jet brunette to chestnut. It was a crapshoot, they said, how it would come back.

As she was deciding on which $500 wig to get, I told my sister that she would never put it on, and she gave me a weird look. I said it again—you know you'll never wear this thing. She held it up the way people hold wigs, raising it to eye level, twisting her wrist, her fingers spreading the nylon mesh inside, and she looked at it some more. It'll be bandannas and maybe hats, but not this. *No way,* I said. She looked back at me. Of course she went ahead and ordered it, since it was insurance money. When we left the wig store, Heidi wondered about how her hair would come back. Curly, she said. She wanted curly hair.

When I came home for Christmas, she was in the hospital, closing out the first round of chemotherapy. She was on the seventeenth floor, up high, near the top. Once I had taken a walk around, certain things I'd never considered became apparent. For instance, all the cancer patients are on a single floor. The chemicals are administered via a port-a-cath, which must be surgically implanted under the skin of the chest. Also, chemotherapy isn't just a single chemo administered via a flat standardized therapy, but a cocktail with any number of toxic fluids topped off by the lone constant—an antinausea drug. Save a guy in his early twenties, she was the youngest person there by a long shot. That's the one thing I had thought about.

I slept on the couch next to Heidi's bed that night. Nurses were in and out, monitoring levels of dripping bags, checking the connection at her port-a-cath, looking at LCD displays that resembled boring video games. Despite their careful and genuine attentions, they brought about a rough night's sleep. I woke up a couple of times; she probably didn't sleep. *Thank you,* I kept hearing her tell the nurses. *Thanks for your help.*

As I walked around the seventeenth floor, I saw many of the patients. They moved languidly in loose clothes, mostly pajamas (Heidi took to old, soft flannel shirts, since the buttons gave easy access to the port-a-cath), and they had in tow mobile IVs that looked like tall, thin, metal coatracks, with bags of liquid swinging where the coats should have been. I made eye contact with many of them, and they had a strong look. There were a few, dispirited, who glared at the floor as if searching for a ledge they could continue over, dragging the coatrack to some deep welcome end; these few already were gone. But the others I couldn't believe. Every look was so vibrant, with a big, brimming heart behind it.

That's when it hit me about cancer. Everybody's always asking what he or she can do. They show up, they bring food and books, they drop off flowers and Bibles, the requisite courtesies that maintain the requisite distance. But it's the other way around, really. The patients are doing everything for you. They bring you in. They throw that strong glance your way, and you know that all you must do is treat them as ever you have before.

Hair disappears, weight rises and falls and shoots up again, IVs plug in and pull out, nausea ebbs and boils. But there is still your sister or brother or your friend, who expects you—*wants* you—not to switch the mood to dire just because that's what people do when others are sick. This underlying simplicity hit me, and my chest swelled a little; I was happy and sad. I breathed deep and went back into my sister's room. I swept a small swath of blond hair off her pillow and put it inside my book. I understood, just a little, what my place in this was. Or maybe I didn't understand it so much as feel it somewhere that I knew counted—right where my chest had just swelled. It seems that, save the very few who want to drag their IVs to a welcome end, those who get cancer are the only ones who can handle it. They're going through it, not you. You're going through something different. You watch the great ones shine; you get to be near them. Like light exposed to a prism, you are transformed.

Families come around, stay around, bring meals, the circles under their eyes like deepening bruises. Yet you can tell that everything under their skin is alive and full, held together by this person in bed whose hair sticks to the pillow. And there are the visitors. They make hesitant eye contact, and they reach their hands out and say: *How are you?* It's emphatic, inevitably, not at all like a question. And the reply, that steady voice: *I'm OK.* She grips the visitors' hands back. That assured and assuring gaze, which wouldn't once be framed by a wig. *I'm OK,* she says. *How are you?*

Friends and Neighbors (FANs)

As I lay in the hospital after exploratory surgery on my "likely benign" tumor, a lifelong friend of mine came in to check on me and seemed all too serious. This was odd: He and I had probably had about two serious conversations in the twenty years we'd known each other.

So he comes in and sits down on the bed next to me with a real sour expression. I'm lying there reveling in a cocktail of opiates. Josh leans in and looks at me for a second and says, "Why didn't you tell us?"

"Tell you what?" I say.

"That it's cancer."

"Well, because I didn't know until just now. Doctor!"

Yeah, he was the one who broke it to me without knowing I had been sedated when the biopsy test came back. It was hilarious. And now I have something to make fun of him for—for the rest of our lives.

—Chris Simpson

You'll quickly realize that Friends and Neighbors (FANs) fall into four general groups:

The I Know Yous

Show us somebody who plows through the bad news and treats you just as you've always been treated, and we'll show you the greatest of FANs. There's an art to balancing compassion and keeping it real, and the best FANs get it. They don't require much discussion, because with them it's easy going post-diagnosis and during (and after) treatment. They're supportive and understanding, but don't let you pull the cancer card without good reason (unless they benefit as well, like getting to the front row of a concert).

The Poor Yous

These guys don't really expect you to leave your bed—ever. They look at you with pity, talk in hushed tones, and are the most likely to launch the dreaded question: "How aaaarre you?" (This question, we should note, is "dreaded" only when the asker's implication is something along the lines of "You know you can confide in me and only me how monumentally shitty everything is.")

Poor Yous think they're being exceedingly understanding when their every word and gesture indicate one thing: *awwwwwwwww.* They'll start the shower running for you, they'll run to the store to get you stuff to eat and drink. They'll pretty much do anything for you, since they operate under the assumption that you can't do jack shit for yourself. Though this sometimes will indeed be the case, it's every bit as certain that it's a downer to assume that it always will be.

You'll find more Poor Yous in your closer circle of family and friends. Their concern for you is genuine, so don't go off on them just because they're going overboard. Make clear to the Poor Yous that you haven't really changed into an incapacitated being, but you might need their help sometimes—and you'll tell them when that happens.

The Lucky Yous

Still others think that because you have more free time now, you're the perfect babysitter/

leaf raker/carpool driver/etc. They think they're treating you as they always have—you know, not cutting you any slack—but they lack the compassion that indicates that they really get what you're going through.

Lucky Yous likely aren't part of your close circle of family and friends, so your interactions with them, though occasionally annoying and often touchy, won't take up much of your time or energy. Blow off any unreasonable requests they toss at you, but don't get angry at their ignorance—being angry sucks up too much of your much-needed energy.

People with Cancer (PWCs)

The rarely sighted, the proud, the snow leopards of Planet Cancer. With a little effort, you should broaden your social sphere to include some PWCs. You can find other young adults with cancer online, via local support groups or by attending a retreat like the ones Planet Cancer puts on (with travel scholarships!). (See "Resources" for ways to connect.)

You may be wary of PWCs at first, especially if you've never seen or talked with another patient or survivor your own age, but trust us—you want to find these people. They get it. You don't have to fill in the backstory. They laugh at the same things you do, and you don't have to censor what you're saying because you're afraid it might be awkward or uncomfortable.

Remember that it's better to have people around you as you fight cancer than not to, so even if you encounter FANs who haven't a clue, it's usually better not to lash out at them. Smile and laugh—at them, with them, whatever—and hope they come around for the ride.

Managing Information, Well-Wishers, and Info-Seekers without Going Crazy

- **Name one person as Chief Information Officer** (CIO) and make him or her responsible for getting updates out to family and friends. You cannot and should not handle every single phone call and e-mail!

- **Start a blog and send the page link** to family and friends to keep them posted on your progress. (Go to http://myplanet.planet cancer.org.) You or your CIO can maintain the page.

- **Record your outgoing voice mail message with a daily or weekly update.** You can include a sentence saying how much you appreciate the support and warn them not to expect a return phone call. Then screen your phone calls and only answer the ones you really want to.

- **Make a list of things that you want or need help with** (be as concrete and specific as you can: driving you to the doctor, babysitting, grocery shopping, mowing the lawn, doing your laundry, cooking dinner on Wednesdays, etc.). Post it online or hand it over to a Chief Support Officer (CSO), who will connect volunteers with tasks. Direct people who want to "do something" to your CSO and the wish list.

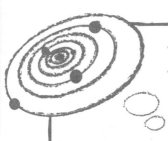

Dispatches from the Planet

When I was first diagnosed, I wrote a letter that described what was going on, what my treatment and prognosis were, and told everyone how I wanted them to respond (and how *not* to respond). I sent it to just about everyone I had ever met in my entire life. I didn't want word getting out through the grapevine, and I didn't want anyone holding pity parties for me. The response was tremendous! I got sunglasses, cartoons, hats, funny pictures, jokes, and plenty of encouragement that helped me through my treatment, many from people I hadn't heard from in years.

—*hl1994*

When I got out of the hospital, one of my neighbors said, "Since you're not doing anything right now, why don't you head one of the committees next year?" Hello, I'm fighting for my life here! I was still on home IV drugs and starting radiation, not to mention my entire abdomen had been cut and I couldn't so much as sit up by myself. But yeah, let me run right out and start decorating the neighborhood for the holidays.

—*Chrisan*

My best friend dropped everything, drove three hours, and surprised me on my doorstep with a box of Audrey Hepburn DVDs. She kept track of when my appointments were and called me after almost every one to see how things were going. Now, we're closer than ever.

—*J*

I had a thyroidectomy, and when people asked if they could visit me after surgery, I said I would only accept visitors who came bearing flowers or scarves! I now own lots of scarves and turtlenecks to cover up the scar.

—*Kate*

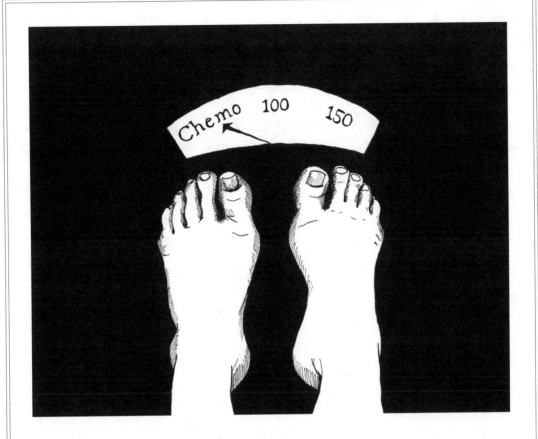

Top 10 Ways to Cut the Cancer Conversation Short

10. Yeah, well, I was getting sick of my haircut, so I figured, Why not?

9. You should see how many presents I got.

8. Chemo is a great way to lose weight.

7. People are a lot nicer when they think you might die.

6. It was a perfect opportunity to get caught up on all my soaps.

5. Yeah it sucked, but look at this badass scar!

4. How else do you think I got into college?

3. Now I get to wear this trendy yellow bracelet.

2. I don't really remember it. I was too drunk most of the time.

1. I didn't have anything scheduled for that year anyway.

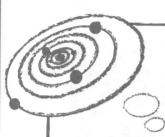

Dispatches from the Planet

I know it seems simple, but how you tell people "the news" is everything, you know? If you present it in this crappy, pathetic, defeated way, then you'll get those crappy, pathetic, defeated faces looking back at you. But if you talk about bustin' it up, you get the opposite! I love it!

—Cassidy

The whole "who do I tell, what, when, and how" question (I guess that only leaves out where and why) is tough. Personally, I've decided that at this point, my cancer experience makes up too much of my adult life to leave someone in the dark about it for very long. Like chemo itself and so many other things in this world, two people can respond totally differently to the statement "I had cancer," but I think that it's a good start.

It took me a while to realize that, without any preliminary explanation, what to me was a funny story could end up dropping jaws and opening eyes, especially if I was asked to explain the circumstances. Going at it from the other direction (telling people I had cancer first and letting things go from there) seems to give me a chance to judge reactions before pushing into deeper territory. And while that first statement is still scary, on the whole I've gotten more positive responses to it than negative.

—Kyle

{ Some Helpful Things to Know about Interacting with PWCs }

by Theresa Gambaro and Kate Thaxton

There are rules for social interaction that apply to cancer patients and survivors—rules that, if followed correctly, can help us avoid the pitfalls that threaten our sense of well-being and our friendships, and that inadvertently place us, shuddering, on the periphery of mainstream society.

Theresa Gambaro writes:

1. Avoid making comments about our appearance. We all want to hear that we look good; I can't tell you what I wouldn't do to once again experience the workplace sexual harassment of my pre-cancer life. That said, we have had physical changes—some bad—and we are self-conscious about the physical differences (real or imagined) that we now have. I have been told innumerable times by well-meaning friends and family that I look so much . . . better. It's true: I do indeed look better than I did bald and retching into a bucket. I do indeed look better than I did lying in a hospital bed white as a sheet with a tube coming out of my neck. It's just useless information.

2. It feels natural to end all of your conversations with cancer survivors with a resounding "Good luck to you!" Don't say it. Hearing this over and over can cause extreme anxiety, as luck has betrayed us in the past. Our relationship with luck is very complicated; the very term "cancer survivor" suggests that we are both lucky and unlucky at once.

3. Bringing up your personal religious convictions is a potential quagmire. Tread lightly around faith-related topics, and don't impose your beliefs.

4. Don't ask us, "How long have they given you?" Ever. The only applicable statistic for anyone, really, is 0 percent or 100 percent, and it's easy to calculate: If your heart is beating, it's the latter, which is encouraging. Still, I respectfully enjoin you to relinquish your curiosity or camouflage it more appropriately. Or use Google.

> { Avoid pity compliments: I despise these. "At least you look cute in hats." }

Kate Thaxton's counsel:

1. Don't assume my type of cancer: A lot of people assume I have breast cancer—I guess that's because I have breasts. I get that a few times a week and still have yet to come up with a witty response.

2. Depression: Despite the stockpile of anxiety meds, I don't think I'm depressed. I have the occasional meltdown, but for the most part, I think I'm in a good place. Maybe that's the

denial talking, but whatever the case, for you to assume the worst regarding a cancer patient's emotional state doesn't help anything.

3. Avoid pity compliments: I despise these. "At least you look cute in hats." Thanks, but I looked cuter with hair. Just a bit of advice: Try to avoid using "at least" when giving a compliment.

4. Gifts: Don't assume that presents need to be more profound or meaningful because I have cancer. I still love chocolate and jewelry.

5. Hair loss: I went a year without losing my hair. Don't make the assumption that someone wearing a "F*ck Cancer" shirt doesn't have the right to wear it because she has a full head of hair.

6. Restaurants: Please don't make me pick the restaurant because you think I have an aversion to a certain food. I hated making the restaurant choice before cancer, and I still hate it. I'll let you know if something doesn't sound good.

7. Cancer questions: Don't assume that I don't want to talk about cancer. If you're comfortable talking about it, then so am I. Talking about it actually provides some sense of comfort for me, so don't be bashful—if you have any questions, just ask.

Dating

It's not exactly something to look forward to, meeting someone during treatment: "Hey, I'm thirty-one, I've got one nut and might be infertile, and I probably have toxic chemicals in my body at this very moment. Let's do this!"

—GAVIN

Why get all worked up on the first date if I may not even like them enough to waste the emotional energy it takes for this reveal?

—PLUMPDN

Suffice it to say that for most people, cancer is not a huge turn-on. And if it is, well, you probably want to watch out for those people. If you're in treatment, you probably aren't at the top of your dating game physically, emotionally, or mentally. This fuzziness can be distressing, but a valuable lesson here is that, for now, the focus probably needs to be on you.

Post-treatment, the eternal question is "When do I tell?" (And the corollary: "How do I tell?") Disclosure is a huge issue in the young adult cancer community. Chat rooms and message boards dedicate a lot of acreage to discussing these questions, and we'll address them below.

During treatment, though, don't sweat disclosure. That said, having cancer or a history of cancer can be a great personal litmus test, saving you much time trying to determine whether a potential partner is worthy of your valuable time and energy. After all, if they can jump in the fight with you or express suitable awe and admiration at your survivorship—they just might be worthy partners to come along for the rest of the ride.

Top 10 Pickup Lines for Cancer Patients

10. A night with me is better than chemo.

9. Is there heparin running through my veins or is it hot in here?

8. I've got a scar shaped like a hickey. How about giving me a real one?

7. What's your diagnosis? I'm a Cancer.

6. It's not just my head that's bald, you know.

5. Is treatment lowering your BBT (basal body temperature)? Because you sure are cool.

4. Hey baby, let's go back to my place and compare scars.

3. You must have lost all your hair, because you are smoooooth!

2. Let's go back to my hospital room: You play doctor, I'll play nurse.

1. Is that a chemo pump in your pocket or are you just happy to see me?

Bonus: A cancer personal ad: "Bald druggie seeks SO for hookups, incisions, and full body scans. I'm used to getting 'special' treatment, but my port is always easy access."

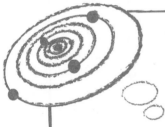

Dispatches from the Planet

You know, just be honest. Even if some people flee as a response. At least you know. What you've also gotta know is that just because you had cancer doesn't mean that you're gonna be single. You're just gonna have a different outlook and different needs. Start with the nurses in your hospital :).

—*peterframpton*

The idea that cancer is a skeleton in my closet or that it's my darkest secret makes me very angry. Cancer has been an intense, personal, and in the end, net positive experience for me, and every time I have to deal with someone who feels that cancer is a skeleton to be hidden, I have to remind myself that some people just aren't worth trying to have a relationship with.

On one hand, I've got a very different view of life than most twenty-three-year-olds, but because I was either very sick or at least on treatment from the age of eighteen through twenty-two, I missed out on a lot of dating opportunities. The "old" part of me doesn't want to waste time on something meaningless, but the "young" part of me just wants to go out and have some fun. Doesn't make for easy dating, what with the young guy and the old guy getting into it.

—Kyle

I think the misconception is that survivors are single because the "c word" scares people off. I think it's myriad other factors we (survivors) have in common that make us less likely to pair up for the sake of pairing up. I had a boyfriend when I was diagnosed but had to break it off halfway through because cancer is an experience that makes you reevaluate the way you are living your life.

Since I'm pretty confident at this point that cancer isn't going to kill me (anytime soon), my new greatest fear is settling! I'm twenty-six and have married friends, some more happy than others. I'm saying now that I'd rather be alone than unsatisfied with whomever I end up with.

—KayCee

A guy friend of mine (who is a cancer survivor also) and I were at a party. A girl was talking to him about running a marathon, and he leaned in to me and said, "Little does she know I only have one lung!" We both started laughing and making jokes about it. The girl just didn't get it, just felt sorry for my friend—the last thing he wanted/needed. There is a disconnect, and I think it would be great to date someone who understood and could also laugh at the insanity of it all.

—Jessica

I feel like as soon as I mention it, it sets off a hundred thoughts in the other person's mind. Whether their reaction is ultimately good, bad, or neutral, there is always that awkward silence as they try to digest this word. I think that most people have a certain imagery they associate with a cancer patient. They have to reconcile that with the person they see sitting in front of them, and that can be difficult.

Some people will say that you are still you, only more. And some can't see past the word "cancer." It's a very important part of who we are and I think it's a good part. It's made us all stronger, wiser, and more compassionate people. So whenever and however you decide to mention cancer to a partner, don't be ashamed or afraid to do it. You can say it with all the nonchalance or calm you can muster, but cancer is a big deal to most people. If the other person isn't capable of handling it, then they just aren't. And I believe that all of us deserve someone who can love every single part of what makes us who we are.

—Shanti

I don't think you can point to any one time to tell people. It's different for every person you deal with. But if you keep explaining it on the first date and don't get a lot of second dates, that's a sign that it's too heavy a topic for #1. For a lot of people, #1 is just about seeing if you like how the person laughs and whether they can talk about things that don't bore you to sleep—exchanging lots of historical details is for later. For someone who has not had a similar experience themselves, "It's affected every part of me" is very intimidating.

—Steve

Top 10 Reasons to Date a Cancer Chick

by Leigh Tomlinson

10. I'm a cheap date—probably won't be eating much.

9. No need to take me to expensive restaurants because, if I do eat, it will probably come right back up.

8. I can be ready in a jiffy—only have to wash crevices.

7. Recreational drugs are paid for by insurance.

6. Commitment-phobic? I'm your dream girl.

5. Great in the sack. (That one would have made the list either way—but really more so now because I'll often be in it!)

4. You'll always be the pretty one.

3. Strangers will really think you're special and extra compassionate.

2. You will get first dibs on all my possessions, and since I'm shopping to cover my fear, you'll come out waaay ahead.

1. With all my wigs, I'll be a different girl every night.

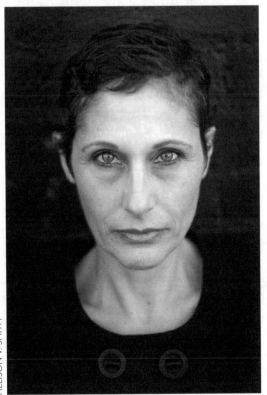

ALLISON V. SMITH

Guides to the Planet

Leigh Tomlinson passed away while we were putting together this book. Her strength, her spirit, her oh-so-twisted sense of humor, her quick smile—all of Leigh will continue to represent the best of Planet Cancer.

{ Putting Yourself Out There on Planet Cancer }

by Tracy Maxwell

By the time I had at least two to three inches of hair back, I decided I looked normal enough to not have to deal with the question of whether I was a lesbian or a cancer survivor on the first date, and I put myself out there. I started trolling the personals on Craigslist—a first for me. I have done the online dating thing before, but always the services that required payment, and usually I had been overwhelmed by the number of incoming e-mails. This time, I decided to do the choosing myself rather than wading through responses.

There were about five guys who seemed smart enough, funny enough, and normal enough. I e-mailed all of them. All of them responded, and most of them kept e-mailing even after photos were exchanged.

I guess there was a pretty good connection both ways with one guy. We are having our third date tomorrow night, and I still haven't revealed my cancer status. Why? I don't really know. I like him. I feel comfortable with him. We've even talked about health care several times. It just hasn't come up.

How do you tell someone that you know wants kids (because he mentioned it in his ad) that you probably won't be able to have them because you are now one ovary lighter, and chemo poisoned your eggs?

I try to put myself in his position. How would I react if someone I was dating told me he had had cancer? I'm sure I would wonder how long he's going to be around, and whether it's worth

getting involved with someone who may have a shorter life expectancy and may well get sick

> While no one will probably ever list cancer on his or her Match .com profile—unless it's an astrological sign—it should be something we are comfortable talking about and dealing with.

again. It's one thing if you're already in love with someone and he or she gets sick, but would you choose to get involved in that scenario? I will never forget my grandma's advice—she was a nurse—when I mentioned in high school that I had a crush on this guy who had diabetes. She ran down all the problems related to that chronic disease and told me I would be better off liking someone else.

While no one will probably ever list cancer on his or her Match.com profile—unless it's an astrological sign—it should be something we are comfortable talking about and dealing with. After all, more and more young adults are being diagnosed with cancer these days—there are one million survivors under forty at last count. There is a whole movement serving this segment of the cancer population, and more awareness is being raised about the unique needs of this group. The myriad dating issues I have mentioned will be faced by a significant segment of dating-age people in the future. I guess that means I need to practice my reveal.

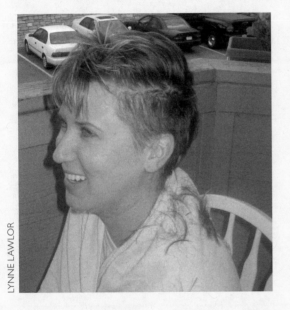

LYNNE LAWLOR

Guides to the Planet

Tracy Maxwell was diagnosed with Stage IIB granulosa cell ovarian cancer in 2006 at age thirty-six. She lives in Denver, Colorado, where she serves as the executive director of Hazing Prevention.Org, a nonprofit organization she founded. She writes a monthly column called "A Single Cell," published on divinecaroline.com, about the challenges of dealing with cancer as a single woman.

{ Dating and Disclosure }

by Sage Bolte, ABD, LCSW, OSW-C
oncology counselor, *Life with Cancer*

Dating and knowing when to disclose your cancer history can create a lot of anxiety and fear around being rejected. Before you begin to explore dating during/after cancer, it is important to get comfortable with yourself as a survivor, with your new limitations, scars, hair and skin changes, or changes in the way you perceive yourself—both positive and negative.

It is important that you are comfortable in telling your own story and comfortable with what you have to offer in the relationship before you begin to date. If you are not comfortable with your own story, in your own skin, in your own ability to date, then someone else may find it difficult to accept you (this is true whether a person is a survivor or not).

> It is important that you are comfortable in telling your own story and comfortable with what you have to offer in the relationship before you begin to date.

If you are uncomfortable with the changes in your body, spend time reconnecting to your body and finding things about it that are good and attractive. To get comfortable with yourself and your body during/after cancer:

- Offer yourself positive affirmations every morning in the mirror, such as "I accept that my body will work with me and not against me in the healing process," or "I believe I have much to offer in this life and in my relationships." By starting our day with positive thoughts, we influence the way we see ourselves and possibly the way others see us. (We cannot vouch for anecdotal reports of the affirmational merits of affixing a Steven Seagal poster next to your bathroom mirror.)

- A common self-esteem-building exercise is to stand in front of the mirror every morning or evening and find three things that you like about your body (this could be the curve of your nose or the color of your eyes; it doesn't have to be something sexual at first).

- As you get better, you will feel better. That improvement will help with feeling more comfortable in your skin.

- Find a counselor who can help you address your feelings.

How to Disclose and Date

- Be comfortable with your own story so you can share it at your own pace. One of the best ways to get comfortable is to role-play with a friend. Act as though you were on a date, and practice ways to tell your story.

- There is no right or wrong amount of time to tell or not to tell—is there a way to slowly disclose or tell all at once? Choose ahead of time what is right for you regarding the right time to disclose.

- Put yourself in the other person's shoes: How would you react? What would you want to know and not know initially?

- Include your story in your online profile or online social networking page if you want it to "be out there" before you meet.

- Seek out online groups that connect you to people who "get it."

- Take advantage of survivorship conferences and camps—maybe Mr. or Ms. Right will be there!

- As stated above, make sure that you have done your own work and become as comfortable as you can in your own skin so that you are comfortable with someone else's touch.

Significant Other / Caregiver

We had a cutoff of when we could talk about cancer: 8 p.m. If we had stuff to talk about, it got written down for next day. This was really helpful for me.
— AMANDA

We feel strongly that Planet Cancer's denizens aren't only People with Cancer (PWCs). There are the significant others and caregivers as well— whether they have cancer or not, these spouses, parents, siblings, and pathologically dedicated friends are present for all the ups and downs. The old saw for when parents punish their kids applies here too: It hurts the caregiver every bit as much as it does the patient, sometimes more.

The following intro was written for us by an authority on this subject. Sarah Wenstrand was a cancer partner alongside her husband, Mike Moore—his back was host to the most badass biohazard tattoo of all time—for twelve years until he died in 2007. Thanks for dropping some knowledge, Sarah.

{ Things to Keep in Mind as a Caregiver or Significant Other }

by Sarah Wenstrand

If you're fortunate enough to have someone in your life who'd do absolutely anything for you and you'd return the favor, count yourself lucky. When life deals that someone a cancer diagnosis and he or she comes to cash in that valuable chip, however, you've gotta decide whether or not to pay up.

If you sign on, it will be much more than a superficial commitment. You either sign on or sign out. Otherwise you're an obstacle for supporters who are all in. So take stock of yourself, listen to your heart, figure out what you can offer, and communicate that to the (possibly fragile but not yet broken) newly diagnosed. This makes it easier on everyone and, if not right away, then let's hope that down the road the person will appreciate your honesty.

With enough fortitude to stick it out, you'll embark on a world that offers new challenges, heartbreak, and rewards daily. Not to mention all the complimentary soda crackers and lots of time to catch up on outdated pop culture mags! (Sign you up, right?)

As a cancer partner you'll be expected to perform many roles, including battle buddy, receptacle of entirely too much information (think "bowel movement frequency"), family contact point, researcher, medical coordinator, and general gofer. All this responsibility is yours, in addition to maintaining your own sanity.

But wait. There's more! Combining this partnership with the dynamics of your existing relationship as mother, father, sibling, distant cousin, fiancée, spouse, co-parent, or other role is when the real party ensues. Two or more of those designations and you have the potential chaos of: young adult children moving back in with caregiver parents; blissfully ignorant lovers smacked into reality; concurrently being soft shoulder and meds-monitor; or taking leave from your job to care for your children and your partner. Cancer could have you undertaking totally unexpected interactions, like sperm banking with your boyfriend or having waaaayyyyy too many conversations containing the word "breast" with your father-in-law.

Well-meaning but vague offers from those on the periphery ("If I can do anything to help, just let me know") will at times infuriate you. Solution: Turn those empty platitudes into action items. People do want to help; they're just not sure of the role you and the rest of the key players are comfortable with.

Beware "diagnosis amnesia." Before cancer interrupted our lives, we were successful businesspeople, creative souls, confident parents, fun-lovin' twentysomethings, etc. & etc. You might forget some of these traits because your world just got dumped upside down. Treatment could put enormous pressure on you to maintain everything else in life to allow your partner to focus on fighting to live.

To that end: As someone who is caring for someone else, you'll need to streamline taking care of numero uno (that's you), or you'll both suffer. Self-nurturing could be as simple as making sure to wax your eyebrows each month (after all, chemo hasn't stunted *your* follicular function) or as immediately necessary as power walking laps around the infusion center.

You'll be attempting to gauge your own mental and physical health in addition to that of your care-

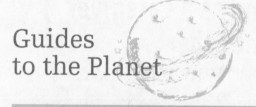

Guides to the Planet

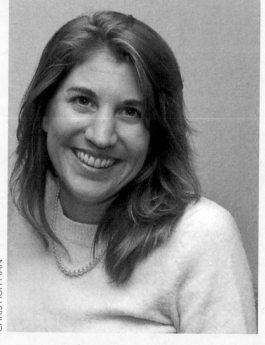

CHRIS HUFFMAN

In a time before daily use of e-mail, search engines, social networking, and even mobile phones, Sarah Wenstrand graduated college the same week her long-distance boyfriend, Mike Moore, was diagnosed with Hodgkin's lymphoma. Her caregiver initiation was composed of cross-country relocation (twice), the sperm-banking process, chemo, and marriage—all within the first eight months. While Mike concentrated on fighting cancer for the next twelve years, Sarah served as medical coordinator and personal photographer of her husband/muse, who died on March 6, 2007. Since Mike's death, Sarah has been committed to raising awareness about the issues faced by young adults with cancer and their partners, which has included working as an ambassador for Planet Cancer's advocacy initiatives to cancer centers. She is also participating in and facilitating Writing as Healing workshops at her local cancer center. Her future plans include using her experiences as a caregiver and as a young adult surviving spouse in the area of patient navigation.

recipient. Sometimes you're expected to do so with the know-how of a trained nurse. You wish you could order up a Matrix-style download of knowledge.

Some caregivers dive in headfirst, hunting their great white whale, and others take a more cautious toe-dip approach. Whatever method works for you and the diagnosed is what you should embrace: Go back to what you know, seek to learn what is necessary, and enlist the expertise of professionals for the rest. It may take some time to figure out, but at least you get to laugh amidst blundering failure. After all, this isn't brain surgery. (Warning: Brain surgery may be involved. Odds are slim that you'll be expected to perform it.)

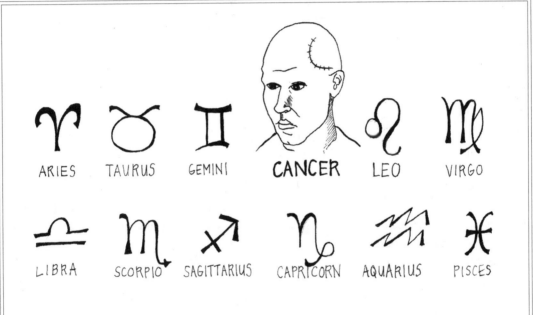

ARIES   TAURUS   GEMINI   CANCER   LEO   VIRGO

LIBRA   SCORPIO   SAGITTARIUS   CAPRICORN   AQUARIUS   PISCES

Top 10 Worst Responses upon Learning Someone Has Cancer

10. Other than that, how's it going?

9. This isn't going to affect my career, is it?

8. I guess there's no need to quit smoking.

7. There are easier ways to build character, you know.

6. Oh, my aunt/cousin/grandfather died of that same cancer!

5. Be sure to wear clean underwear.

4. You'll save on shampoo.

3. Cancer . . . before or after Aquarius?

2. Whatever.

1. It's always about you, isn't it?

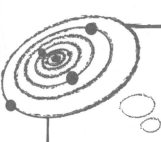

Dispatches from the Planet

I can talk to him about anything at any time. I don't mean just talking about cancer. I literally mean anything. On chemo week, he mostly loses his memory. We still talk even though I am going to have to tell him everything again by Friday. Just knowing that he is there (even if his memory isn't) makes getting through this so much easier. My simple solution for supporting your loved ones is communication.

—Mpaquet

The way I see it, cancer happens to the couple/family, not just the individual. Every aspect that changed for my husband in post-cancer life also changed for me. My job experienced setbacks, my parenting suffered, finances were tricky, etc., etc.

We needed each other to get through his cancer. I can attest that treatment days were horrible for me, watching my loved one go through that. I ate and ate, because it was the only action I had that felt like I was doing something. It wasn't only watching him get injected, but also knowing what was to follow that seemed so frightening.

While my husband lived very much in the moment, I had to always live a few steps ahead of him to make sure our lives were held together. When treatment days came, I had to be prepared for everything, not knowing what the next moments would actually be like.

What saved me was having a friend who was my guardian. Sure, she cared about my husband, but she mostly cared about how I was doing. Still does. She was the person that I went to for personal support, drinks, mindless chatter, a breakdown, fits. I went to her when I simply had to be strong for my husband.

—Andrea Jenkins

Though he would never trade in me and our son, going through this with a spouse and child adds another set of issues. I know it seems the grass is always greener, huh? He has said to me several times, "You don't deserve this" and "You never imagined this when you married me." He expresses some guilt in having other people involved. Of course, I never regret my life with him and would never change one thing about it (except cancer, of course). Bottom line is, it sucks either way.

—ajenks22

In **April 2002 I was diagnosed** with Hodgkin's lymphoma at the ripe old age of twenty-nine. After my initial surgery to biopsy my tumor, I had to have another surgery one week later to have a port placed in my chest. Since this was my second surgery in two weeks, I was in a real hurry to get out of the hospital that day. I was still a little loopy from the anesthesia, and I really wanted to get out of there. As my husband was putting my shoes on for me, I told him, "You're a regular Ted Bundy." He looked at me and cracked up laughing. He said, "I think you meant to say I am a regular Al Bundy" (the character from the TV sitcom *Married with Children* who sold shoes for a living). We both cracked up. That's when I knew that in order for us to get through the experience, we were going to have to laugh a lot.

—Joanne Vought

A Caregiver Survival Guide

by Lisa Tehan

What to Do

1. **Learn to be patient.** Nothing happens quickly at the hospital. You know you're in love when you can sit at the hospital for eleven hours and still have things to talk about when you get home. On the other hand, learn when it's time to put on the gloves and fight to make stuff happen at a pace your partner needs (see No. 4).

2. **Ask if your significant other would like help managing medications** (pickup, drop-off, doses, making sure they are taken). Don't assume he or she can keep track of this information.

3. **Think of ways to make the hospital more fun** by bringing in video games, magazines, movies, etc. Have date night in the hospital room.

4. **Advocate!** Sometimes people don't know what you and your significant other need unless you ask.

5. **Become friends with the social worker and the nurses.**

6. **Carry around a notebook** to write down all of your questions to ask at the next doctor's appointment.

7. **Pay attention to details.** Your life will be simpler if you learn how long certain procedures

take, what time the nurses change shifts, if visiting hours are enforced, what numbers mean in terms of blood counts and vital signs (see "Demystifying the Complete Blood Count Test" in chapter 2), etc.

8. **Take walks together** around the floor, the hospital, and the neighborhood when you're at home. It is good exercise for both of you and a good time to talk. Appreciate your alone time together without hospital interruptions.

9. **Find people who can relate to your situation.** The Internet is a great place (www.planetcancer.org!) to get support. Most people our age have no idea what it's like when your life becomes about cancer instead of about school and going to parties. These forums and chats can make you feel much less alone.

10. **Cuddle.** A lot.

What to Get

1. **Something that allows you to write down everything** (appointments, scans, blood counts, medications, chemo schedules, consults, etc.). Have a dry-erase board on the wall, and back it up with a notebook or spreadsheet, etc. (See also "Hey Left Brain: Some Jobs for You" in chapter 2.)

2. **A really good blender** to make smoothies when mouth sores and nausea begin.

3. **A subscription to Netflix or Blockbuster online.**

4. **A lot of hand sanitizer.** Require people to use this before they come in the door.

5. **Books on CD or e-books**—for you to have something to focus on as you drive to the hospital, and for your significant other when he or she is too sick or tired to read.

6. **Gatorade and Ensure or Boost.**

7. **Winter hats.** Being bald is cold.

8. **A knee pillow** to make sleeping more comfortable for your significant other.

9. **A lot of books, Sudoku, and crossword puzzles.**

10. **A blog or Web site** to keep family and friends updated so you won't have to call everyone every time there is something new to report.

What Not to Do

1. **Sleep at the hospital every night.** You may think you are sleeping there, but you can't sleep well if you are listening to IV alarms, nurse call buttons, and vital signs.

2. **Let sick people near you or your significant other.** This includes people who even think they might be getting sick!

3. **Let people tell you that you need to go on vacation.** We all want to go on vacation, but leaving your significant other at home can make it more stressful than relaxing.

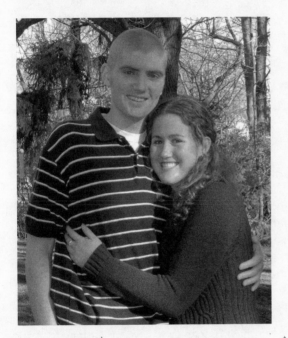

4. **Treat your significant other differently.** You may be taking care of him or her, but you are still a team.

5. **Make decisions for your significant other without asking for his or her opinion.**

6. **Try to do everything by yourself.** Ask parents, siblings, relatives, friends, and coworkers to help you. People want to help!

7. **Avoid talking about cancer, death, and fear.**

8. **Only talk about cancer, death, and fear.**

9. **Stop taking care of yourself.** You will get sick if you become run down, and sick people can't take care of sick people.

10. **Feel guilty** for wishing he or she had never gotten sick.

Guides to the Planet

Lisa Tehan's fiancé, David Russell, died of acute lymphoblastic leukemia in 2008, at age twenty-three. Lisa cites knitting as her therapy since David passed, along with time with her family and friends and helping other young people affected by cancer. David's passions, Lisa writes, were family and music—he wrote music and played the piano and trumpet. He also raised money for the Leukemia and Lymphoma Society and the American Cancer Society.

At Your Beck and Text: The Importance of Not Being Consumed

by Sarah Wenstrand

As a cancer partner, you'll be on call so much you'll feel like a doctor (among other reasons). Luckily, technology has improved over the past dozen years, and we can use that to our advantage in the quest for balance in a life that is otherwise dedicated to someone else's health and survival.

When my then-boyfriend, Mike, was diagnosed in 1995, we had no such newfangled gadgets. I'm not talking carrier pigeons here, but the pinnacle of contemporary communication when Mike started treatment was "the brick." When I decided to move from California to North Carolina to be there for Mike during his treatment, Mike overnighted the behemoth cellular albatross cross-country before my mom and I set out on the five-day road trip.

The brick wasn't used for daily contact, however: It was too expensive! So, when I would leave the apartment during that first six months of Mike's treatment, the brick was a staple in my trunk. It was a gamble, me leaving him, but we were still young, optimistic, and invincible.

After our marriage and return to California, we decided I needed a pager. My job kept me away from the phone, so it enabled me to do something important for myself. I felt like a drug dealer. We devised a numerical code that was so infrequently used that I'd freak out anyway and have to hunt down the nearest pay phone pronto.

So, what does this have to do with you, the modern caregiver, now that we have instant communication at our fingertips? There were times when I was out of reach of Mike and my immediate responsibilities to him. It might have been a tinge worrisome, but it was necessary for me to have that time "off." Although now we have the convenience and peace of mind afforded us by technology, as a caregiver I think it may hinder our ability to self-nurture when we have the opportunity to, similar to people who are expected to check work e-mail and voice messages while on "vacation."

I'm not saying ditch the phone and leave your cancer partner in the lurch. What I am saying is that, in the context of your partnership, find ways to enable yourself to be out of touch for small periods of time. This may require you to enlist the help of willing family or friends, notify nurses about alternate emergency contacts, or, if your partner is able to be alone without worry, simply come to an agreement not to call you during this period of radio silence. Whether you need an hour to do yoga, get out for an afternoon in the sunshine, or spend two weeks in Australia (dare to dream), the peace of mind that comes with knowing you won't be interrupted is very valuable to someone who otherwise has to be on alert.

An added bonus: You might even be missed by your partner. And missed not because your partner "needed" you for something, but because he or she was lonesome for your company. Who am I kidding . . . maybe your partner needed a break from you too.

Becoming the Primary Caretaker, Ready or Not

by Amber Wadey

In May 2003 I noticed a mole on my husband's back was growing and looking a little strange. We'd been married for about five years, and I was working on a degree in health education. You'd think I might know a thing or two about the ABCs of skin cancer, but we were twenty-five and felt a little invincible. Making doctor appointments was not a priority.

Eventually, I was buying two-inch square bandages and waterproof tape to cover the mole, which was growing so quickly that it had ulcerated. The lab results came in the mail in a wrinkled envelope that looked as though it had a rough time getting into our hands. I opened it and read the results: "potentially serious malignant melanoma." How serious could it be now that it was gone?

Chuck called the dermatologist's office to figure out our next move, which was to see a surgical oncologist. That was the last appointment I let Chuck go to alone. Just before Labor Day weekend, almost four months after first noticing that ominous mole, I came home to a terrified husband who had heard only one thing from his surgical oncologist: She was going to do some tests to see if it had metastasized and said something like, "If it's spread too far, there's no point in operating."

We were given several treatment options ranging from don't do anything and hope it doesn't come back, to a year of interferon therapy, to intense bio-chemotherapy. This was when being the primary caretaker became overwhelming. Suddenly everybody was looking to me to become a melanoma "expert," to be Chuck's researcher and advocate, to make his care my number-one priority. It was the last thing I wanted to do.

I didn't want my life to change. I didn't want to be the wife of a cancer patient, I didn't want to arrange sperm banking, and I didn't want to be the one to make treatment decisions. I didn't want to feel pressure to drop out of school, I didn't want to fill out short-term disability paperwork, and I certainly didn't want to have to consider what my life would be without him. But I did all of those things.

I decided to approach our oncologist with one question: If it was his son, what would he do? Chuck was young and otherwise healthy, and this cancer was aggressive, they said, so we should treat it as aggressively as possible. Chuck's parents did not agree with this plan, but we'd made up our minds. Five doctors, five months, and five opinions later, Chuck was being admitted to the hospital for his first five-day round of bio-chemotherapy.

Now we're more than five years out. Chuck is cancer-free. We have a beautiful daughter. We all wear hats and sunscreen, and we'll never take a vacation to Hawaii. She'll see a dermatologist regularly, and Chuck will probably be the one to make her appointments. We never wanted to be cancer experts, and we know our story isn't unique. But we feel confident about the choices we've made, and we count ourselves among the lucky. I know my husband would second that.

{ There's a new normal
for you; you've just got to
figure out what it is. }

What Now?

When I was finished with treatment, I felt like my life just suddenly started right back up again without me. Everything went "back to normal," only I wasn't normal anymore. It takes time to digest these big lessons.

—SHANTI

We're all gonna die someday. I think that those of us who get cancer as young adults, though, have to face this reality earlier than most. It's not easy facing the reality of the grim reaper, but it's also not lip service to say that this realization leads to real and earnest living during the time we've got left.

—MRPAUL

As I neared the end of my chemo treatments, I pinned a big photocopy of a bald photo of myself on the wall of my hospital room, labeled "Pin the Hair on Me." I hung a bag underneath filled with different colors of yarn, and made anyone who walked in the room— doctors included—put on a blindfold, pick out a piece of yarn, and try to pin it on. I figured it would predict as accurately as anything else what color my hair would grow back. And where!

—HL1994

You can leave Planet Cancer in many ways. You've done your time in treatment, but you know cancer will always be a part of you, even if it's disappeared, burned away like a clingy morning fog. There is a new normal for you; you've just gotta figure out what it is. Maybe you're eager to leave the Planet—you want to jump into your old life like your favorite shoes and run back to living cancer-free. Perhaps you've put off having a family and you're eager to start.

Or perhaps you want to pursue a new direction you'd never considered before cancer set up shop in your body. You know, do something new—trade in the IV for hiking boots. Or you want to retreat for a while, marshal your thoughts and energy and figure out exactly what cancer has done to your life and what it all means to you.

Or, finally, your exit from Planet Cancer might mean an exit from the world, with the good-byes and finality that never really seemed as if they were coming.

Maybe the fact of leaving itself isn't so much on your terms. But how you leave the Planet damn sure is. Read on.

Transition and the New Normal

I get annoyed when people say, "Well, at least the hard part is over." Is it? I suppose. But sometimes I feel like now is the hard part. It's as if you're thrown into the deep end of the pool for the first time and expected to know how to swim.

—ALLIE

Take baby steps. Try to find something "normal" that you enjoy and perhaps have neglected since your diagnosis. I started heading back to the gym—slowly. I took walks when I needed to clear my head. I started heading to my coffee mornings with friends again. Little things. As much as you can handle.

—RUNNIN DONNA

I had a hard time at first going back out into the world, seeing people again and especially having no hair. I found that I had to just jump back in, and screw the people who stare or have a hard time dealing with it. I don't have time for their issues!

—NESSALOU

One of the first things you have to know after you're done with treatment is that you're likely not going to bounce back into being the same person in the same life you had before your diagnosis. In fact, you might have some periods that oddly seem as difficult as your toughest times during treatment.

This weird parallel universe is often called the "new normal." On the outside, things might look just like your "regular" life B.C. (Before Cancer): Your hair is growing back, you started work or school again, your days no longer revolve around blood draws and whether you pooped or not and whether that poop looked like something spilled from a nuclear reactor. But on the inside, everything has shifted, and it can be hard to recalibrate.

Your priorities are different. Maybe you can't understand why people seem so shallow. They want you to be happy and "back to normal," but you may be feeling tired and not up to par (for a long time), you worry about recurrence, you're dealing with late effects, your job doesn't seem important anymore, you want to do something "meaningful," and so on.

Plus, along with your cancer survivor medal (ha—we wish!) comes all the requisite baggage of regular tests, scans, and the responsibility to monitor your own health, relaying complicated medical information to new doctors and viewing new health developments in the context of what is now a much more complex medical history.

Remember this: All these abnormal feelings *are* normal. You'll have moments of clapping yourself and everybody you know on the back, jumping back into the world and giving it a big hug. But you probably won't feel like that all the time. And that's OK.

You've finished your treatment and are merging back onto the highway of life. You can actually stay up all day and maybe even into the night, your hair is growing back, scars are fading, and you can blend right in with all the noncancerous people around you.

Finishing cancer treatment can feel a little schizo, actually. You want to leave cancer and everything that goes with it far, far behind. But the thought of losing the security blanket of frequent checkups, blood work, and regular oversight is pretty much terrifying. Rest easy. There are things you can and should do to make the transition off of intense medical care into the rest of your life feel much less like being punted off a cliff with no parachute.

The first thing to consider is that you know your body better than anyone. Period. The medical professionals conduct scans and tests, sure, but much of the time they follow your lead and the information you give them. So trust yourself

Too Young to Die,
Too Old to Survive

by Shanti Parmelee

We are the last of a new generation

Balancing on the point of a needle

Bled of our life and then given another

artificial and hollow to make our own

We are the first of old incarnations

Forged by mustard gas and fire

Tempered by anvils that leave surgical scars

Precision damage from smart bombs and smarter drugs

We are the leaders of a damaged nation

Our temples ransacked but our spirits remain

Open wounds expose our open hearts

X-rays reveal our bones of steel!

We are an exercise in concentration

Mind over matter not matter over mind

And Soul over mind and above everything else

as Soul returns to this smoldering land

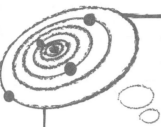

Dispatches from the Planet

I just had my second clean PET scan a few weeks ago, which means I can breathe easy until July. I live my life in three-month increments now, which is an odd feeling that I'm not sure that "regular folks" understand.

—*Jen Singer*

Lord knows this whole experience has changed me for the better. My problem is: All the friends that supported me through all of this seem to have just gone back to "business as usual." I don't even talk to them anymore because I feel like they think things are back to the way they were. Well, they're not. I'm a different person and need help rebuilding my life.

—*Cereal Killer*

During my last treatment, my nurse said she hated that I had to go through this at such a young age—I was twenty-five when it began but turned twenty-six during the experience—but that I would appreciate things more than other people. Nothing could be more true.

—*Haley Mellert*

When I was sick and in treatment, I waited for the day I would be finished. Finished with being devastated inside and out,

and hope to God it all worked. That day came on February 27. What am I waiting for now?

—*Denny*

I finished treatment six months ago, and with a handful of scans/tests, PET, and even a colonoscopy (original diagnosis was nasopharyngeal carcinoma Stage 2B). I felt like my overly protective doctor was keeping one of my feet firmly planted in the life of a patient, as I was trying to get my other one into the land of the living, or so I call it.

Now I find myself having good and bad days. I was always a high achiever, successful, focused. I find myself overwhelmed easily. The most common things:

- I feel pressured to attend events, and I can't decide what to do.

- I don't want to talk on the phone. People leave voice mails, I don't check them, and the box fills up.

- Can't multitask: I get overwhelmed easily.

- I have trouble fixing meals and prioritizing.

Of course all these things are on my worst days. I have very good days also, but I just feel a general sense of being in a rut. This could be career-related also, as I think being out of the loop of the normal grind has caused general boredom, which has led to a bit of depression/ anxiety.

The other thing I think about is whether or not I've gotten "it"—you know, that big realization that we're supposed to get once we've beaten/survived cancer. It's like, what am I doing with my life? Did this enormous thing in my life really change me for the better, and am I taking advantage of it?

I flip-flop from not wanting to think/talk about it, to feeling like cancer was the best thing that happened to me, to wanting to tell anyone and everyone that I had cancer.

—Denny Tu

---

and your instincts and stay in tune with your body. And if you have some false alarms or over-reaction for a while ("My head aches! I know I drank twelve margaritas yesterday, but I bet it's a new brain tumor!"), well, that's OK. Eventually you'll level out and not page your oncologist five times for every new ache and pain.

Next, realize that—congratulations!—you are now on the map. You have been tagged as someone whose every health issue deserves a little bit of extra scrutiny. So if something unusual does pop up, the likelihood is that you will catch it early and tackle it fast.

The next consideration is a little more challenging: You are going to be on this map for a long, long time. Meaning: the rest of your life. Your non-cancer friends don't think twice about whether they have a primary care doctor or if they got their Pap smears this year. You, on the other hand, have an additional burden of responsibility to monitor your health on an ongoing basis. Cancer is in your rearview mirror, but the ripple effect continues: You want to be diligent about watching for possible recurrence, and you want to also be mindful of long-term side effects as a result of either the cancer or the treatment.

Here are the most important things you need to remember as you begin this new journey of long-term follow-up care:

- **When you finish treatment, ask your doctor for a treatment summary outlining your diagnosis and the treatment you received.** Make multiple copies so you can hand them over to every new doctor you see. Believe it or not, you will forget the details of this ride you've been on, such as specific drug names, but that doesn't make them less significant.

> You have been tagged as someone whose every health issue deserves a little bit of extra scrutiny. So if something unusual does pop up, the likelihood is that you will catch it early and tackle it fast.

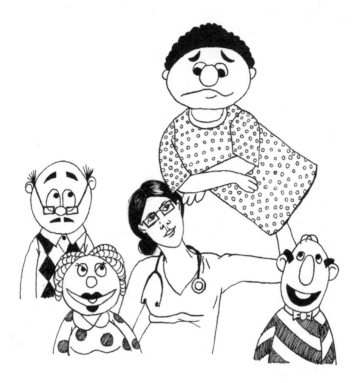

Top 12 Responses to Enduring a Colonoscopy

(From an unnamed gastroenterologist, who claims these are actual comments made by patients while he was performing colonoscopies.)

12. Take it easy, Doc, you're boldly going where no man has gone before.

11. Find Amelia Earhart yet?

10. Can you hear me now?

9. Could you write me a note for my wife, saying that my head is not, in fact, up there?

8. You know, in some states, we're now legally married.

7. Any sign of the trapped miners, Chief?

6. You put your left hand in, you take your left hand out. You do the Hokey Pokey . . .

5. Hey! Now I know how a Muppet feels!

4. If your hand doesn't fit, you must a quit!

3. Hey, Doc, let me know if you find my dignity.

2. You used to be an executive at Enron, didn't you?

1. Are we there yet? Are we there yet? Are we there yet?

- **Also ask your health-care team to provide you with a survivorship care plan,** outlining the long-term side effects you might be subject to, as well as what type of screening tests you should request and how often to get them. The University of Pennsylvania and the LIVE**STRONG** Foundation offer an online tool that generates a plan based on your particular diagnosis and treatment at www.livestrongcareplan.org.

- **If you move, find a doctor as soon as you get there, if not before.** If you're recently out of treatment, get your oncologist to refer you to a colleague in your new town. If you're further out of treatment, a good primary care doc should do the trick.

Maybe it is a giant pain in the butt, and maybe it doesn't seem fair that you have this extra responsibility, but being the guardian of your own health is something we all have to do eventually. Just consider yourself a trend-setter.

Last thought to keep in mind: Going to the doctor does not give you cancer.

Avoiding follow-up because you don't want to know what's up with your strange cough only causes you additional distress as you deny your suspicions and fear. Stick with regular follow-ups, and if something odd crosses your radar, get in there and figure out what's going on. It will either put your mind at ease or clarify your suspicions, in which case you can get moving on a new action plan to take care of business.

Going Back to Work

I used to be such a go-getter type person, but now it seems like I don't do anything. Maybe I am still fatigued from the treatments or something, but now I just make it to work when I drag myself from bed, and when I am there I just don't want to do my work and will pretty much do anything to avoid doing it. It is really unfair to my employer that I am not getting much done, and I feel like such a lazy piece of crap! The brain needs time to catch up. I just kind of did what I needed to during treatment, and now, when I am supposed to be getting back to "normal," my brain just spins.

—LAB

When you're working somewhere and diagnosed, it becomes apparent pretty quickly if your employer falls among the good guys or the creatures of the dark. You either get played and screwed over, obstacles at every turn, or you're supported without question or qualm.

Post-treatment, you're either putting the time in to readjust to your old job or you're pounding the pavement in an effort to get a regular paycheck again. Like any relationship, you're not sure what you're signing up for with a new employer until you commit. You might get hosed, and you might not. Read on for some info about what your prospective employers have a right to ask and know about you and your history.

> **Scanxiety:** The feeling in the days leading up to a follow-up scan that, no matter what test you are about to undergo, it will inevitably show that you have cancer again.

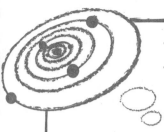

Dispatches from the Planet

Basically, "normal" is a subjective word. You may want to stop putting expectations of this "normalcy" on yourself, because it is added pressure. I too feel like nobody gets it. That's because they couldn't really understand unless they've been there, and it's frustrating, I know.

You can't just put everything in the past and be normal again. I mean, the experience changes us psychologically as well as physically, so there really isn't any going back. You have to see it like this: The same way an adult can't go back to seeing things the same way they did as a five-year-old, neither can we. Cancer survivors are enlightened in ways others can never be, so we can't return to "normal," because we are so much wiser now. Trust in your newfound sense of judgment as your "new normal."

—Cee

When I finished treatment, I thought I'd feel this enormous sense of relief and that all the pieces that got tossed all over the place would come back together and life would go on. Not so much. The time after treatment was harder for me in many ways than treat-ment itself. I stopped connecting with my fellow citizens of Planet Cancer, since I thought I wasn't "supposed to" need to anymore.

Well, "supposed to" does not apply when you're thirty-four and diagnosed with rectal cancer. Once I realized that, I went back to the Planet and it was the best thing I could have ever done. I went on the Planet Cancer 25-40-year-old Retreat a year after I finished treatment, and it was so great to be among "my people." They helped me realize that it was OK to still need to be a citizen of Planet Cancer. I'll leave someday, but I will always have a stamp in my passport from Planet Cancer.

—Carrie Morse

Long-Term Follow-Up

I went to a new doctor to get a physical, and when he was checking downstairs, he said I was missing one of my boys. So I pretended to freak out and told him I didn't know. Ha ha! I told him then that I had had testicular cancer. He is still my doctor.

—Brad

{ What Can Your Employer Legally Ask about Regarding Your Health? }

by Kyle Steuck

It's possible that having battled cancer and come out on the other side has instilled in you a confidence borne from a new perspective. You're ready to go into a job interview and knock it out of the park. What's an interview, anyway, after undergoing more than a year of chemo? Even if this is the case, interviewing after battling cancer can be intimidating for a different reason. Much like meeting people after a cancer diagnosis, we have to weigh the benefits and risks of what to say about the cancer experience, how to say it, when to say it, and whom to say it to.

By law, employers are not allowed to ask during an interview any questions about health, disability, medications, or past illnesses. If you are interviewing with someone with HR experience, that person will know about these restrictions and will usually steer clear of asking anything that might be illegal. However, employers are allowed to ask questions that are directly related to their business, including those related to your ability to do the job and any gaps in your résumé. Confused yet? Some examples:

- What were you doing between June 2001 and May 2002? LEGAL

- Have you ever had an illness that forced you to miss work? ILLEGAL

- Are you currently taking any prescription drugs? ILLEGAL

- Can you perform the duties required for this position (heavy lifting, driving, etc.)? LEGAL

It's also illegal for employers to ask for a medical evaluation before they offer you a job. After the offer, they can ask for a medical evaluation if it's required for everyone in that job category. And after any evaluation, an employer cannot take back the offer unless it directly affects your ability to do the job.

So be prepared—your health may come up during an interview. Most potential employers are going to steer clear from asking any illegal questions about your health. A brief, true, and uninformative description of your "time off" should suffice.

Even after you have the job, your employer must keep any medical records in a separate, confidential file. Discussing your health with a supervisor isn't necessary, although you may have to reveal some details to the HR department. This information must also remain confidential.

What to Say If They Ask about That Strange Gap on Your Résumé

Below, we've channeled some sage advice from the online career counselors at Cancer and Careers (www.cancerandcareers.org) on how to handle questions in a job interview about gaps on your résumé:

Keep in mind that it's very common for individuals to change jobs, to step out of the workplace for personal or family reasons, or to go back to school. So if you're asked about gaps in your employment history, be ready with a short, clear answer that

> **Bottom line: The focus should not be on cancer, but on the future and what you have to bring to the table.**

doesn't go into detail about the difficulties of your cancer treatment. Then redirect the conversation with a question of your own about the employer's needs. Some examples:

"I took some personal time to rethink my career and brush up my skills, and that time allowed me to refocus. I'm excited about using my skills to add value in a firm such as yours. Can you tell me more about _____ [this one sounds good, but don't go there: your extremely favorable policies toward cancer survivors]?"

Or you could try being direct yet positive: "I faced cancer and won. I'm proud to say that I am a survivor. I learned a lot from my experience; it has made me appreciate what I can contribute to the world. I'm eager to make a difference in a role such as the one we are discussing today."

Bottom line: The focus should not be on cancer, but on the future and what you have to bring to the table. Decide how much or how little to reveal about your illness and recovery, and roll with it. Think through your own situation, assess your own comfort level in discussing your health history, and craft a short, positive answer that focuses on what you have to offer a potential employer. Just like in your recovery, focusing on the future and the possibilities for making a contribution can generate excitement not only in you but in future employers.

Celebration

I finished treatment, heard the "R" word—remission—and promptly got tatted again!
—MARCUS

You finished treatment! Yahoo! What now? The options are endless. Have a big party and invite your friends from far and wide. Travel someplace you never thought you'd go. Jump out of an airplane. Play Scrabble next to the fireplace. Walk the dog. You can do whatever you want—and that's the key thing to remember.

While many people come out of treatment with a burning and praiseworthy desire to "give back" in some way, don't feel pressure to start a foundation, volunteer with cancer patients, or "raise awareness" if that's not your thing. Planet Cancer member *1knocR* put it eloquently after reading a feature in *CURE* magazine (a fantastic resource) called "Why I'm Not Climbing a Mountain":

"[The author of the piece] . . . talks about how he doesn't need to prove anything after finishing treatment. His friends, and some rude acquaintances, seem to expect him to do something. I feel the same way, that people expect me to do something. I do do something. I work, I eat, I drink, I sleep, I shop, I walk my dogs, I travel. What else should I be doing? Don't get me wrong, I applaud the survivors that run marathons, participate in Relay for Life events, and climb mountains! But that is not me. I want to do whatever I want to do. Cancer did change me and make me aware of the way

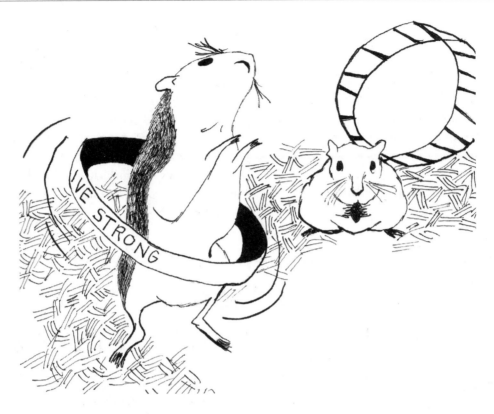

Top 10 Uses of *LIVE**STRONG*** Wristbands

10. Even your gerbil needs a hula hoop.

9. Use one as an emergency car fan belt.

8. Stick in front of teeth and behind lips; make scary faces and frighten small children.

7. Use four wristbands to suspend yourself from the ceiling of exam rooms after the nurse has left, thus avoiding unpleasant procedures or just scaring the living hoo-ha out of your doctor.

6. Make trendy '80s earrings.

5. Slap one on your drink at parties to avoid accidental "shares-ies" germs.

4. Keep your pant leg up so you don't get grease all over it while biking.

3. Diamond rings are so twentieth-century—try a LIVE**STRONG** wristband for your engagement.

2. Shoot at other patients to incite saline bag fights.

1. The latest in tourniquet chic!

I was, and the way I wasn't. But I don't need to prove anything. I went through the eating right, no caffeine, little red meat. I felt limited. Surviving cancer is about living!"

Celebrating is personal. Keep that in mind. But whatever else you decide to do, be sure to take at least a moment to pat yourself on the back and savor this milestone. You earned it.

Family Planning . . . Finally

So you're thinking about starting a family. Whether you've just finished treatment, have waited the more-or-less requisite five years, or are many years out, be aware that cancer may still have a ripple effect on this most important of decisions. If your cancer or treatment has impacted your fertility, you may have to consider alternatives such as in vitro fertilization (IVF), surrogacy, or adoption. There's nothing that points to the future more than having a family, though, and if you're thinking about kids, it's a sure sign that you're moving on from your treatment experience and looking ahead in a positive direction.

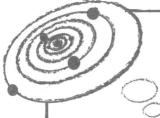

Dispatches from the Planet

Testicular Cancer: A Haiku

Had seminoma
And yet I still joke and laugh
I must be half nuts

—Geoffrey M.

Cancer Woman symbolizes all women with cancers. The flowers represent tumors. She has a mediport. Her hair is falling out, but she is still beautiful, strong, standing, facing forward, and hopeful. She is a survivor. This is one of the hardest paintings I have ever attempted, as I was trying to show pain and suffering, while also showing beauty and hope at the same time. I don't think I could have painted it unless I had gone through the illness myself.

—Sarah Dees

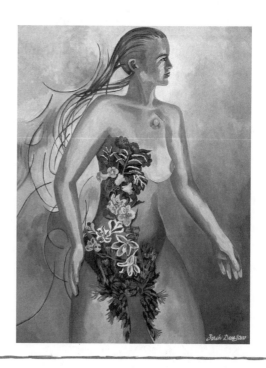

Tattoos

Some survivors choose the tattoo as a way to (indelibly) memorialize their cancer experience. Talk with your doctor first to make sure your blood counts and immune system are fully kicked in before you go under this new kind of needle. You might get some antibiotics from him or her to take as a precaution too.

Tattoo Idea #1: Your patient number.

Tattoo Idea #2: The food that didn't make you nauseated during treatment.

Tattoo Idea #3: An ichthys (the fish that you see on all those bumper stickers).

Tattoo Idea #4: A phoenix.

Tattoo Idea #5: A zinnia (represents friends who are gone).

Tattoo Idea #6: Go to Miami and get whatever tattoo you decide on at Miami Ink.

Tattoo Idea #7: Biohazard symbol.

Tattoo Idea #8: A syringe over the scar where your port was.

Tattoo Idea #9: A chamomile flower (energy in adversity).

Tattoo Idea #10: A cedar tree (healing, protection).

Tattoo Idea #11: An apple tree (magic, youth, happiness).

Tattoo Idea #12: A cherry tree (rebirth).

Tattoo Idea #13: A willow tree (realizing your dreams).

Tattoo Idea #14: A poplar (courage).

Tattoo Idea #15: Cancer ribbon in your cancer's color (www.choosehope.com lists all the colors). Put diagnosis date underneath.

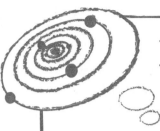

Dispatches from the Planet

You can take the summer off. You can create work you love. You can do anything you want. It is too bad that so many of us need a catalyst to do just that. I'm glad I had one, but I want to tell you not to wait. Do what you want to do now! If you don't know, figure it out. Someone once said the two most important questions in life are: Who are you, and what do you want? Figure out the answers to those questions and you are way ahead of most of the people on this planet.

—*Tracy Maxwell*

I think I always enjoyed life before my cancer, but I really enjoy it now and really take my time when I'm doing special things. Another thing: I started a list of places I'd like to go, and I've already crossed out a few. There are a few places I want to go with my fiancé, yet there's places I'd like to go with my mom. They are not all extraordinary destinations either, some as simple as going to Graceland in Memphis with my mom, which I can happily say we have done and I've crossed off my list.

—*Kelly Cain*

What it's really like to . . .
Consider Alternative Avenues toward Parenthood

by Samantha Eisenstein Watson

When I was first treated for cancer at age twenty-one, I remember briefly asking my oncologist if I should consider freezing eggs (without really having an understanding of what that would actually entail), but as soon as he said I didn't have time—that it was more important to start chemo ASAP—I dropped the question. When I was diag-

nosed again at twenty-three and told I would have to go through a bone marrow transplant, I was more concerned with survival than I was with babies. It just wasn't in my frame of reference.

Eight years later, do I wish I would have done something proactive to preserve my fertility? Maybe. But I can't know whether or not delaying chemo to freeze my eggs would have prevented me from being here now to make the decision. What I do know is that my husband and I want to have a family, and we are faced with an overwhelming number of options—none of which I would have imagined I would someday have to consider.

This past year, we began by researching both fertility options (egg donation and surrogacy were our two choices) and adoption (both domestic and international). My first step, though, was to mourn the loss of my fertility—something I never really allowed myself to do, and something that is certainly an ongoing process. I never wanted pity throughout my cancer treatments, and since then I have tried to keep looking forward. But I did realize that the loss of fertility was an important blow to my identity as a woman.

We are raised with the assumption that someday we will bear children. Society expects us to. Between the trendy maternity clothes and the unending pictures in magazines and TV shows of glowing pregnant women, pregnancy almost becomes an industry in itself. We are made to feel as though of course we want to have children. But language matters. I realized that "having a baby" was not necessarily the same thing as "being a mother." And, after much soul-searching, I realized that I could be a mother—even if I had to take a road off the beaten path to get there.

For both my husband and me, information is key. We both feel a need to make informed decisions (maybe because he has a very practical, logical brain, and I am a self-proclaimed control freak), and so once we decided that we wanted to be parents, we went ahead full-speed in gathering as much information as possible. To start, we researched adoption agencies in our state, found fertility doctors with experience in working with cancer patients, and considered the many countries from which we could adopt.

With regards to adoption, we were forced to deal with important questions about race, ethnicity, and age, and had to think hard about the role of birth parents and the differences between closed and open adoptions. With regards to fertility, we had to weigh the risks that my health history might provide with my desire to physically carry a child, or my husband's desire to have a child genetically related to him.

I am incredibly lucky in that my husband is the most supportive, loving man I have ever known. He truly doesn't care whether we have a baby that has his genes or not and would be happy with any baby that is handed to him—whether in a hospital or in a foreign country—so long as my health is protected at all times. We are both exceptionally fortunate to have supportive families; as this will be the first grandbaby for three sets of grandparents, they are more excited about being grandparents than they are concerned with where the baby comes from or what he or she looks like.

We also spoke to as many people as we could find about their experiences and gained a great deal of very useful information. Parents were very open and willing to share their stories, and they answered all of our questions—no matter how blunt—and tried to address our fears.

The difficult part, for us, was that everyone we spoke to was on the other side of this monumental decision. What was missing were conversations with people in this very same stage: would-be parents grappling with the innate desire to "have a child" and, at the same time, the emotional pull toward adoption. In retrospect, I wish we had sought out more channels through which we could have connected with other couples—whether affected by cancer or not—making these same decisions. I think it would have alleviated some of our frustrations and validated many of our concerns, and I think it would have been tremendously helpful to share resources and information with others either a few steps ahead of or behind us.

Ultimately, we learned that we had to come to a place where we were comfortable, because that would translate into the best decision for the child—rather than feel as though we should adopt from a certain country or are supposed to have a child genetically related to at least one of us. We are still uncertain about which path we will take, but we know from our experience so far that this journey will require patience, flexibility, and determination, no matter which road we go down. We will try to remember to get off this treadmill once in a while to cry, laugh, yell, and scream—because at times this process can be unfair, frustrating, amazing, and exciting, and it's important to take care of ourselves and make sure we are getting the love and support (most importantly from each other) that we need to keep moving forward.

It is exciting to know that the end result of any of the options we choose is a baby. Our baby.

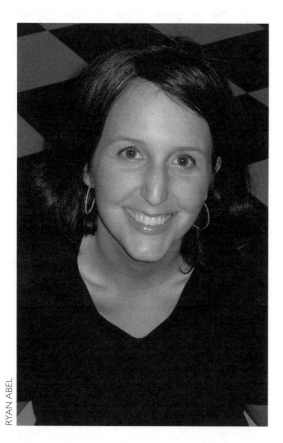

RYAN ABEL

Guides to the Planet

Samantha Eisenstein Watson is a two-time young adult cancer survivor. Diagnosed with Ewing's Sarcoma in December 1999 and subsequently with secondary Myelodysplastic Syndrome in April 2001 (for which she underwent an allogeneic bone marrow transplant), she co-founded The SAMFund in 2003 after recognizing a void in programs and services tailored specifically for young adult cancer survivors after treatment. An active member of the cancer community and an advocate for young adult survivors throughout the country, Sam holds a BA from Brandeis University and an MBA in Mission-Driven Management from the Heller School for Social Policy and Management. She co-teaches an undergraduate Sociology of Disability class at Brandeis and in her "free time" loves to cook and travel. She lives in Boston with her husband, Adam, and their dog, Bella.

{ Adoption II }

by Dr. Michelle Miller

With chemotherapy, my menstrual cycles stopped and chemo-induced menopause began. Menopause never occurred to me and was never mentioned as a possible chemo side effect by my oncologist, so it went undiagnosed for months. A chemo-induced menopause would "likely be a temporary condition," my doctor said. So, with the promise of a future in sight, Joey and I talked about starting a family once I was in remission and my menstrual cycles returned.

After eight months of chemo and three months of radiation, I was pronounced in remission. My menstrual cycles attempted a return, too, and I was under the care of a fertility specialist. Six months later we learned that my cancer was back. One morning, while packing for a month at the bone marrow clinic, a thought crossed my mind: children. The next day, Joey wheeled me into a fertility clinic. We arrived with the hope that we might store some eggs before the stem cell transplant, but the doctor explained that my platelets were too low to risk an egg-harvesting procedure and that I might bleed to death if my blood couldn't coagulate. He refused to do the procedure.

From the moment of my cancer diagnosis, our dreams to make a family in the old-fashioned way were kidnapped with no ransom note. I was furious at the lack of accountability and insensitivity of doctors to not disclose this information to us a year earlier before cancer treatments began. If my doctors had warned me in advance, I might have cryo-preserved my eggs, possibly fertilized and implanted them in a surrogate at a later date—I don't know—but I would

have had options. I learned how all too common it was for doctors to neglect telling their patients about treatment-related infertility.

I was astounded to realize that bias, belief in cancer myths, and outright discrimination existed in the adoption community. During my telephone inquiries I was candid, at first, about the details of my disease but, routinely, when the word "cancer" was uttered, the conversation was over.

I was sad to discover that, to most of the public, despite decades of advancements in medicine, a cancer diagnosis meant certain death. Yes, I had cancer, but I was thriving in spite of it. Some adoption agencies hung up on me, left me indefinitely on hold, or never returned my calls. "Why would we adopt to you when there are hundreds of couples who don't have cancer?" a social worker asked me. "What if I didn't have cancer anymore?" I asked. "I hardly think that a birth mother will choose someone with a cancer history over someone who does not have one," she retorted. In a few cases the adoption workers I talked to believed that cancer was contagious or that stress from parenthood could reignite cancer in someone who was cured. Some believed that cancer was caused by unhappiness.

Some adoption agencies wanted a five- or ten-year remission before they'd consider working with a cancer survivor. For some people, such a time delay meant that they'd be considered too old according to the criteria set by adoption agencies themselves. Other agencies wanted documented proof from a doctor of a complete cure.

"Are there any guarantees for any of us?" I'd ask. "What's to say that you adopt a child to a seemingly perfect couple and twelve years down the road they get divorced, or are killed in a car accident, or one of them dies of cancer. . . . Does that mean that you didn't do your job?"

In these instances, they didn't hold themselves accountable for unforeseeable events after an adoption was finalized. But, because all adoption workers believe that their primary duty and obligation is to be the advocate for children and birth mothers, the majority opinion was that cancer survivors do not always rank high on the list of desirable adoptive parents. However, a few agencies that I spoke with said that they had adopted a child to a handful of cancer survivors over the years. To those that did, they did not want to be considered a "cancer-friendly" agency. I also knew of many cancer survivors who had successfully adopted, but the fact that I experienced adoption bias at all was something

that I never expected. After all, wasn't having a loving mother with cancer better than being an orphan? Interestingly enough, I discovered, too, that not all cancer survivors disclosed the truth about their health status for fear of adoption rejection. Adoption was certainly possible for cancer survivors, but for someone like me with ongoing cancer, adopting a child was a million-to-one shot.

After so much rejection and emotional trauma, out of the blue, a gift: Our daughter was born on January 1, 2008, at 8:22 a.m., seven pounds fifteen ounces, twenty and a half inches long—a healthy, gorgeous, precious gift from God. The birth parents relinquished their rights in writing forty-eight hours after birth as required by state law, witnessed, notarized, and signed by a judge. We brought our daughter home from the hospital at three days old, and we haven't stopped smiling since. At forty-one years old, I am finally a mother. My daughter is the best medicine I've ever had.

What it's really like to . . .
Be Diagnosed for the Fifth Time

by Glenn Rockowitz

There was something about that dick that I will love forever.

Sure, he was a redheaded, thick-necked, handlebar-mustached ex-con who had done fourteen years in Joliet Prison for assault and armed robbery. And he was a dick. But I loved him anyway.

I loved him because he taught me something. He taught me about the most important something. He taught me about cancer. About its nature and its weaknesses and its pitfalls. About its brutality and its unfairness and its indifference to suffering. But above all, he taught me that the wicked little fucker could be beaten into submission. Or, ideally, remission.

Of course, he had absolutely no idea he was teaching me anything. He was just a chemo neighbor with no personal boundaries and way too many hours to kill. So while I silently prayed for a way out of my grim Stage IV non-Hodgkin's lymphoma diagnosis, I sat and listened to a series of delightful prison rape stories.

One story in particular stayed with me. A dark ritual that the prisoners of Joliet performed on every new inmate as he entered prison. A ritual they affectionately referred to as the Rodeo in Joliet. It worked this way: Every time a newbie was admitted, the general inmate population had an unspoken agreement to let him feel safe, let him feel like everything he may have imagined prison life to be was probably exaggerated.

That period of calm would last three days. And on that third day, a group of the other prisoners would surround the new guy and . . . uh, well, *make love* to him. And not in the robes, scented candles, Kenny G kind of way.

Once that initial lovemaking session was over, they would let the guy stand up and walk away, let him think that the rite of passage was over. Let him think he was now safe to go about his day. But alas, he was mistaken. Because before making it to the other side of the prison yard, the Rodeo would begin all over again.

And while the story didn't strike me at the time as anything other than another horrific tale from my charming leather-skinned chemo buddy, it became—over the course of the last nine years—the perfect metaphor for my fight with this disease.

It seemed that every time I started to feel safe, feel that I'd done my time, feel that cancer's lovemaking with my imprisoned ass was over, I got knocked down again. And every time I got knocked down, it became increasingly more difficult to stand back up. More difficult to get out of bed in the morning and put one foot in front of the other. More difficult to just breathe without fear.

But it's hard. Really fucking hard. Because it's a different kind of fear. It's an ambient fear, an ever-present hum of anxiety. A little like that feeling of

> It's a different kind of fear. It's an ambient fear, an ever-present hum of anxiety.

tipping back in your chair a bit too far and catching yourself before you fall. But it's all day, every day.

Over the past nine years, I have been diagnosed with four different cancers. One of them twice. And the routine is always the same: I go in for tests and I go home and I wait and I wait and I wait and then the phone rings and I pray that it is a nurse or an assistant or a receptionist and it never is. It's always a doctor. And when a doctor calls, it's bad news. Period. I have yet to have one call me and say, "After looking at your CT scans and your blood work, I have to tell you that you have great loafers and a winning smile."

It is a free fall. And it never gets easier. But there is a silver lining. And it's something all cancer patients will tell you, especially young adults: You are now on the map. Now that you're sick, you'll be under surveillance. And the likelihood

WHAT NOW?

of catching anything new at an early stage is far greater. So yes, the Rodeo may continue, but it loses strength with each showing.

When I originally sat down to write this piece, I had planned on closing it with a message of hope and optimism. After all, I had just passed nine months of being disease-free. No scares, no phone calls, no confusing reports, no we-need-to-look-into-thats. But alas, as I was making my way across the prison yard, convinced that I was safe, I was surrounded and knocked down again. It appeared that my remaining kidney—I had lost the other one to renal cell carcinoma in 2005—was starting to fail.

As of this very moment, I don't know where this will go and I don't know what will come of it. Maybe nothing. But I guess that's the point: It doesn't matter. I just need to turn off the Kenny G, put away the scented candles, and stand the fuck back up.

Guides to the Planet

Glenn Rockowitz is a writer, comedian, film-maker, and a four-time cancer survivor. He is the founder of Best Medicine, a nonprofit that provides comedy performances for homebound cancer and AIDS patients. He is currently forming *Change It Back,* a Northwest coalition designed to improve treatment standards for adolescent and young adult patients. His memoir *Rodeo in Joliet* was released nationally on April 11, 2009.

Death—A Fact of Life

I find myself thinking that I know when I'm going to die. I never say it out loud to my family members. I just see and hear about young women with my similar diagnosis and stage, all dealing with metastatic disease, and I know the reality that it can happen to anyone. Hell, cancer happened to me in spite of the odds. It's not a doom and gloom look at things, and that's what I think people around me wouldn't understand. It's just thinking about it, coping. I can't imagine not thinking about it when it has been thrown in my face.

*—*CRISSY

I look at it this way—at least I have a chance to say "hello" and a chance to say "good-bye." Lots and lots of people don't get that chance.

—ANNETTE

That's right. Death is indeed a fact of life, so let's not gloss over it. Once you accept that, it becomes evident that, well, there's a lot to dying. It can be overwhelming for reasons other than being untimely or merciless—there's a lot to take care of. As Annette mentions, the upside (there's an upside?) is that those who know death is coming have a chance to settle their scores and accounts. We'd trade the upside, too, but hey.

Julie Larson, LCSW, young adult program director for CancerCare, which provides counseling, education, financial assistance, and practical help to people with cancer and their loved ones, writes below about how best to navigate dealing with death. Learn more about CancerCare at www.cancercare.org. Thanks, Julie.

Cancer is the leading cause of nonaccidental death among twenty- to thirty-nine-year-olds.

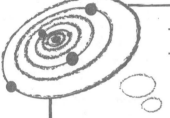

Dispatches from the Planet

Recurrence: Stuck on the Planet

I watched older patients get treatment that they knew wouldn't cure them but could relieve some of their symptoms. There's a quality-of-life balance that can be reached. That may include treatment or it might not, and it's something that can and should be evaluated and reevaluated on a constant basis. I think I'd want to be offered a range from intensive treatment to less aggressive treatment to no treatment in a continuum, rather than with some on-off switch. It's such an individual, personal decision. And an incredibly hard one.

—Kyle

The dumbest thing anyone has ever said to me was over the phone. I called the doctor's office to see if my scans were back. I wanted to set up an appointment to speak to the doctor in person. I was put on hold. Minutes later, a nurse got on the phone and said, "Hello, Mr. Sullivan? Yes, the cancer has returned. The doctor should be calling you in a few days to discuss it."

Just like that. That was how I found out that I had cancer again. For the third time.

"All right, great. Thank you. I will be looking forward to it."

—superfluke

How to Approach Death and Dying

by Julie Larson, LCSW, young adult program
director, CancerCare

It is impossible to face your mortality without stirring up powerful emotions. From the moment you hear the word "cancer," many complex thoughts and feelings may surface. The instinct to suppress these thoughts is understandable. We are often taught to control our feelings and stay positive. But feelings like fear, anger, guilt, or sadness can be important to explore. When you give yourself permission to throw back the curtain and acknowledge what drives your underlying fear, deep sorrow, or swell of anger, you will discover the essence of you.

Death is a natural part of living. I have sat with many people, however, who have been apprehensive about talking about their death—fearful that saying these words out loud will somehow hasten the process. But the tender thoughts and feelings that are tucked inside can give us important clues about that which matters most to you. By facing the reality of your death, you are afforded an opportunity to honor the most vital aspects of your life.

Accepting your own end of life is a process, not a moment. Everyone finds his or her own way in his or her own time. Remember, this process is about honoring your life. The following suggestions may help you focus your thoughts and feelings:

- Consider important conversations you feel you would like to have, and organize your thoughts by writing down the key messages.

- Give thought to whom you would trust to ensure that your end-of-life medical decisions

> **By facing the reality of your death, you are afforded an opportunity to honor the most vital aspects of your life.**

are communicated with and honored by your medical team.

- Share your wishes for what would be meaningful to you and your loved ones at the end of life. This may include preferences regarding having a memorial service and what that service will be like (music, flowers, speakers, location).

- Seek the counsel of a priest, rabbi, minister, or spiritual leader for support around questions and conversations about spirituality and end of life.

- Visualize an inner place of peace and security where you can retreat and find comfort.

- Address unfinished business in terms of your finances and relationships.

- Choose specific personal items to give as special gifts to certain people in your life. You might also choose to give the gift with a note about why you have chosen the item for this loved one.

Hospice Care: It's Not What You Think

Too often, physicians are reluctant to discuss end-of-life issues with their patients, fearing families aren't ready to hear about them. When approached with the prospect of entering hospice, many patients and their families balk at the idea. In fact, the majority of people agree to hospice just days before they or a loved one dies, if ever at all. They feel that even entertaining the thought of hospice means that they've given up and that all hope is lost.

This is unfortunate, because hospice and palliative care focus on pain, symptom management, and psychosocial and spiritual aspects of care so patients can achieve a better quality of life during the time they have left. In essence, hospice gives patients more control over the final chapters of their lives—so they can be free to live until they die, as opposed to dying until they die.

Good hospice care facilities provide:

- Clear discussion between patient, family, and physician about quality-of-life issues

- Pain and symptom management

- Access to daily/weekly in-home nursing care and volunteer support services

- Continued access to cancer treatment such as chemotherapy and radiation for palliative use

- Assistance with end-of-life issues, such as estate planning, wills/living wills, medical power of attorney, and burial plans

- Support for the family in addressing end-of-life issues

Medicare pays up to 90 percent of all hospice services, but private insurance can cover them as well. Hospices are paid per person per day, and the cost increases if the care moves from at-home to an inpatient unit. Also, a patient's home can be considered a long-term care facility. Inpatient care can be at a hospice or a hospital.

Another misperception: There's not a single, huge, grim reaper–type organization that provides hospice care for everybody everywhere. Hospice care is provided by many organizations. Get a recommendation from a doctor or from a trusted nonprofit as to the best options near you. While hospice can be contacted at any point during the treatment process, patients need to be certified by a physician and the hospice medical director as terminally ill, with the expectation of death within six months.

www.lifegem.com: LifeGem creates diamonds out of the carbon from your cremation. Less expensive is to have your ashes sealed within jewelry made to contain it. (Pro: pretty; con: creepy.)

www.memorialspaceflights.com: We had to include it. Get shot into space if you want. (Pro: being in space; cons: littering space, family visits.)

www.soulbursts.com: Have your ashes blown into glass art. (Pro: less expensive than a diamond; con: glass art.)

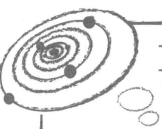

Dispatches from the Planet

Fighting is never a word I would use in relation to cancer. I also do not call myself a "cancer survivor" because it has always sounded wrong to me. I did not do anything exceptional to survive. I did research, worked with my doctors, followed my treatment protocols. Many people do the same thing and do not survive. To say it is just a matter of fighting, or being positive enough, or some such crap, makes death the fault of those who died, and that's just bullshit.

My friend Judy and I had a saying about sadness and anger: "Invite it in for a cup of tea." "Fighting" it was silly and pointless. Yes, we had cancer. Yes, it changed everything. Yes, it sucked. Yes, it brought up a lot of other things in our lives: hopes, dreams, philosophical shit. That was bound to make us sad and/or angry. We lost friends. I eventually lost her. If we "fought" our feelings, our tears, our anger, it just exhausted us, and we didn't feel any better. So, we invited it in for a cup of tea, let it run its course, and then got on with life.

When her death was imminent, Judy certainly wasn't going to fight it. She said the things she always wanted to say and prepared herself for the next big adventure in life.

—*vpiazza*

When I was diagnosed, I made a very conscious decision that my cancer would not kill me, even if I died from it. The moment I gave into it, instead of into the treatments, the moment I let its fear change me for the worse, the moment I let it destroy my hope and my will and my joy, then cancer would have killed me (and it still could). I take this and apply it to everyone else. Cancer doesn't kill us even if we die because of it, if we don't let it swallow our joy.

I'm not a complete optimist, mind you. I accepted when I was scared, in pain, and angry. I owned those emotions. I felt them, but I also still lived my joy.

—*amanda*

{ Leaving a Legacy }

by Jennifer Potter

I didn't meet many young survivors during my treatment for metastatic thyroid cancer. So, I decided to start a social networking group called Young Adult Cancer Survivors of Atlanta. When I started YACS, it never occurred to me that some of my cancer friends would die. They were young and took a kick-ass approach toward cancer. How could they die?

When two of our fellow YACS died in the summer of 2007, it felt as if I had been kicked hard in the stomach. I could not stop crying. The other young survivors in my group felt the same way. We were saddened by the loss of our friends and frightened by the grim reality that it could have been any one of us. It was a huge reality check.

We decided that doing a project in honor of our friends would help heal our hearts. One of the young women who died was an artist, so we painted a piece of artwork through a nonprofit organization called Hospital Art. As we painted, we talked about the two young friends we lost and the wild mix of emotions caused by their deaths. We poured our hearts and souls into that painting.

When the painting was finished, we donated it to the hospital where one of our friends received treatment. We also took a picture of the painting and sent it with a note to our friends' families. It was a great way to honor our friends, support one another through sadness, and give back to the community.

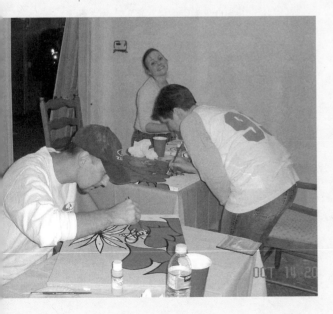

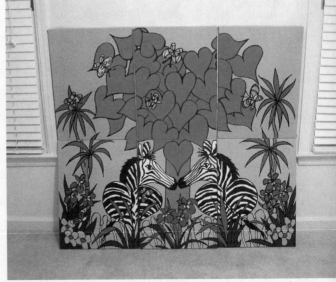

{ A Legacy for Your Children }

by Julie Larson, LCSW, young adult program
director, CancerCare

Talking with your children about death can be challenging. Talking with them about *your* death can seem impossible. Feeling unsure or ambivalent about where to begin and what to say is normal. It is important to remember that children are very tuned into the energy and tone of a home. They know when something is wrong, the situation has changed, and the people who care for them are upset. You are taking care of your children when you find simple ways of being honest and straightforward. They are able to trust you; they have time to anticipate and prepare for what might happen; and they remember that you are available when they feel worried, scared, or sad.

There is nothing more important than letting your children know how you feel. While intense, uncontrolled emotions can be frightening for young children, your honest tears and sadness can also give them permission to release their feelings to you in return. Much of parenting is about communication, and the final messages you give your children can be some of the most meaning-ful gifts you bestow upon them. The suggestions below may help you consider the messages you will leave that will last your children a lifetime:

- Leave messages "into the future" by writing notes to your children for milestones in their lives: the first day of school, Bar Mitzvah/con-firmation, graduation, marriage, birth of a child.

- Create a photo album or scrapbook together of special times.

- Make a video diary or record messages to your children with expressions of love and your wishes for them.

- Keep a journal about yourself. Include memo-ries from your life, qualities about yourself, moments you learned from, or people you cherished so your children can continue to know you as they get older.

{ Life and Death and Life. For Leigh }

by Heidi Schultz Adams, founder, *Planet Cancer*

Essay excerpted from an e-mail dialogue on Planet Cancer.

Hey Heidi, I got home from yoga tonight and opened my e-mail to find that a friend, somebody I wasn't particularly close with but who I spent a week with at Camp Mak-A-Dream, passed away last week. Her name was Holly, and a year ago when we met, she was in treatment, but one of the brightest, spunkiest, hardest fighters there ever was. I am just sitting here crying and I'm so angry . . . it's not that I was close with this girl, but she wanted to live and was a positive-thinking fighter and it just feels so wrong . . .

How do you deal with this knowing so many young adults with cancer? It just makes me feel so mortal. It's like I am doing everything I possibly can, have access to the best possible care and support, but it just kills me because so did Holly.

—*Jason*

Hi, Jason—

Wow. You know how to pull out the tough ones, don't you?! And your timing is uncanny because I'm working through a loss of my own right now that has really hit me hard: My wonderful friend Leigh died a few weeks ago. She was in her forties, a singer and actress with a wickedly twisted sense of humor and a way of making every single person who came into her sphere feel special.

So, let's see if I can bring my half-formed thoughts into something that makes sense, for both of us.

I met Leigh through her boyfriend, Scott Barber, who was our artist-in-residence at some of our earlier weekend retreats. Scott had recurrent lymphoma and died of complications from a transplant. Leigh was diagnosed with breast cancer a year after Scott died. She went through treatment, had a few months of "all clear," then it came roaring back. She fought for the next year and then died on January 5.

I was with her at her home when she died, along with her family, her dog, Happy, and a gazillion friends. It's so weird in those circumstances, when people know what I do. They always say, "You must see this all the time," as though I have some sort of secret insight or password. I never know how to respond.

Yes, I know many people who have died. It is, for sure, an occupational hazard.

Yes, it is painful and raw. Every single time. Sometimes more than others.

No, I never get used to it.

I have thought a lot about dying and death ever since I was diagnosed myself. Leigh's brother gave me her copy of one of the books that I found strangely comforting twelve years ago during my own treatment—*The Tibetan Book of Living and*

Dying—and I find that it is comforting once again as I reread it and mourn her loss.

Her death is not a moment of sadness, grief, and loss, but becomes instead an opportunity and cause for happiness as the instant that she became pure energy and love, and freed herself of the pain of her physical being.

That doesn't mean that it doesn't hurt like hell when I realize, every morning on my way to work, that I can't pick up the phone and call her to check in and bounce Top 10 ideas off her. But I am trying to come to terms with the fact that that's just me feeling sorry for myself.

So how do you and I deal with this reality and go on? Maybe the best response I can give is from a conversation that I had with Leigh after Scott died. I don't even remember whether she had been diagnosed yet or not. She was lost and sad and questioning the point of going on, when someone like Scott—strong, positive, a fighter in every sense of the word—could lose the battle.

I remember that my answer came, through tears, without any thought or deliberation. It was something to this effect: "We go on because Scott would have given anything to be able to do so, and that choice was taken from him. We have that choice, so we choose to go on, and we honor him by living and loving and being joyful and appreciating every single second that we have on this planet. Because he can't."

Personally, I can't default to "everything happens for a reason." It feels like a cop-out to me. Nor can I go down the path of "It's what God wants." Unlike many people whose faith is strengthened in these circumstances, cancer has made me abandon the idea of a personal God up there picking and choosing who gets sick and who doesn't, who lives and who dies.

I think if I believed that, I would get so angry that it would probably destroy me. I have known way too many amazing, positive people who have died, and I have come to believe that their cancers weren't caused by anything but stinkin' bad luck and a bum roll of the genetic or environmental dice.

> We honor him by living and loving and being joyful and appreciating every single second that we have on this planet. Because he can't.

But that doesn't mean I think we are at the mercy of a totally random universe. We do hold a certain amount of control in our hands: the ability to research, to find the best treatments, to do everything we can—physically, mentally, spiritually, and emotionally—to maximize the impact of those treatments. But beyond that we have to realize that every single person brings their own individuality to the experience, right down to the cellular level, and that there is so much we don't know that it is really impossible to make comparisons. We all do the best we can, and that's all we can do. Period.

Every once in a while, when several deaths occur in succession, as they often do, I feel myself getting emotionally "thin." When I'm at home, I have to just close the office and go home to play with my kids. When I was at Leigh's house before she died, I started feeling like this, and I reached out to Dave Marsh, a writer and an incredible mentor of mine who lost his daughter Kristen to sarcoma and is really the whole reason I started Planet Cancer. Here is a portion of his response to me:

But you carry on—I mean, you, personally, Heidi—for the same reason that I do, and Joanne does, and a lot of others, including the best of the doctors and nurses. At its simplest, we do it because we can and because there are so many more people we have known whose struggle didn't work out or did for a while and then didn't, and they need to be honored. . . . What I take from them [cancer patients] is much more immeasurable than what I give. They know the value of life, which is a much more interesting thing, to me, than anything at all about death. So, do me a favor, and thank Leigh as you once thanked me, for reminding you of what the intensity is like when you're in the fight. Leigh has your love, and she gave love to Scott, love of a very high order. She's a winner, not a loser, because if it just boils down to how long we breathe, then everybody's a loser because nobody lives forever.

Dave's so right—there is a certain intensity of life when you're constantly faced with evidence of your own mortality, and only those who have come up against this same evidence can understand it. I would never have known Leigh or Scott or you if it weren't for being in this cancer world. The relationships form more quickly and go deeper faster, because we don't know how long we have, but we do know what's important. And as painful as it is to lose friends, I cannot imagine not having had them, or you, in my life. I have to back off from time to time, because I can't always live on that knife's edge of life and death, but I always return.

So take time to grieve your loss, and then take a few deep breaths, lift your head, and rejoice in the knowledge that this amazing person was and is part of your very living being. I never knew Holly, but I bet that's what she would want you to do.

And now that I've written all this, I know Leigh is chiding me to do the same thing. Up there, shaking her finger at me and saying, "C'mon, precious one. Get a move on."

(Jason died six months after this conversation. He is missed and still loved.)

247

Chapter 1—Diagnosis

American Cancer Society: Treatment Decision Tools

www.cancer.org/docroot/ETO/eto_1_1a.
asp?from=fast (800) ACS-2345 (800-227-2345)

The American Cancer Society's treatment information is legitimate and easy to read. The Web site also includes the NexProfiler Treatment tool, a program that analyzes your own disease information and displays treatment options that might be available to you so that you can make an informed decision along with your doctor.

Anderson, Greg. *Cancer: 50 Essential Things to Do,* Third Edition. New York: Plume, 2009.

Cancer.Net

www.cancer.net

Check out the "Newly Diagnosed: First Steps to Take" section, found under "All About Cancer," for solid information from the medical professionals at the American Society of Clinical Oncology.

Harpham, Wendy Schlessel. *Diagnosis: Cancer: Your Guide to the First Months of Healthy Survivorship,* Expanded and Updated Edition. New York: W. W. Norton & Company, 2003.

Macmillan Cancer Support

www.macmillan.org.uk

An easy-to-understand site covering the cancer basics from our friends in the United Kingdom.

Rosenthal, Kairol. *Everything Changes: The Insider's Guide to Cancer in Your 20's and 30's.* Hoboken, New Jersey, John Wiley & Sons, 2009.

Fertility
Fertile Hope

www.fertilehope.org (866) 965-7205

The go-to resource for every young adult cancer patient exploring fertility preservation is Fertile Hope, now a program of LIVE**STRONG**. Fertile Hope was started by Lindsay Nohr Beck, a two-time young adult survivor of tongue cancer. The organization offers resources and information on cancer and fertility, provides financial assistance, drives research on the impact of cancer treatment on fertility, and educates oncology professionals about the issues around preserving fertility.

Fertility Neighborhood

www.fertilityneighborhood.com

Freedom Fertility Pharmacy sponsors this site, which provides information on infertility, treatment options, financial support, and financing fertility treatment, including financial assistance information.

Researching Your Cancer
American Cancer Society

www.cancer.org

The American Cancer Society is the eight-hundred-pound gorilla on Planet Cancer. It provides help with all aspects of cancer, from call centers to assistance with clinical trials and everything in between.

Cancer.Net

www.cancer.net

The American Society of Clinical Oncology's site of oncologist-approved cancer information. Offers disease-specific information and resources on coping, survivorship, and advocacy and includes a wealth of information for young adults with cancer.

National Cancer Institute

www.cancer.gov (800) 4-CANCER (800-422-6237)

Cancer.gov is the National Cancer Institute's Web site, a comprehensive resource of cancer information including the basics on disease types and all NCI-sponsored clinical trials. The site also has phone assistance and live chat for online help.

OncoLink

www.oncolink.org

A University of Pennsylvania-sponsored, user-friendly site with comprehensive information about cancer.

Steve Dunn's Cancer Guide

www.cancerguide.org

Created by kidney cancer survivor Steve Dunn, this site is "dedicated to helping cancer patients find the best treatment for their disease by finding, and understanding, the best and latest information on their disease." A gold mine for the cancer patient seeking information, including how to research clinical trials, navigate medical databases, and translate research findings.

Misdiagnosis

Federation of State Medical Boards

www.fsmb.org/directory_smb.html

(817) 868-4000

A complete listing by state of medical boards. Most allow you to research doctors and file complaints.

Chapter 2—Getting Your C-Legs
Insurance and Procuring Care

Centers for Medicare and Medicaid Services

www.cms.hhs.gov

Medicare and Medicaid are federally funded programs that are administered by individual states. There are no national guidelines that govern the program, so eligibility requirements vary from state to state. Visit this site to research the benefits available in your state.

Cover the Uninsured

http://covertheuninsured.org/stateguides

A site from the Robert Wood Johnson Foundation providing guides to finding health insurance coverage in every state.

Find a Health Center

http://findahealthcenter.hrsa.gov

An online resource from the U.S. Department of Health and Human Services, Health Resources and Services Administration. This site will connect you to federally funded health centers, even if you have no insurance.

Health Insurance Info.net

www.healthinsuranceinfo.net

A site from the Georgetown University Health Policy Institute offering a state-by-state consumer guide for getting and keeping health insurance.

Patient Advocate Foundation

www.patientadvocate.org   (800) 532-5274

The Patient Advocate Foundation is a national nonprofit organization that seeks to safeguard patients through effective mediation assuring access to care, maintenance of employment, and preservation of financial stability. PAF serves as an active liaison between patients and their insurers, employers, and/or creditors to resolve insurance, job retention, and/or debt crisis matters relative to their diagnosis through professional case managers, doctors, and health-care attorneys.

United States Department of Labor Employee Benefits Security Administration— Consumer Information on Health Plans

www.dol.gov/ebsa/consumer_info_health.html

This site provides consumer information and links on health coverage, COBRA, HIPAA, and much, much more, including how to file claims and appeals with your insurer.

Financial Assistance

Chronic Disease Fund

www.cdfund.org/default.html   (877) 968-7233

Provides prescription co-pay assistance and therapy management for underinsured patients with certain cancer diagnoses.

HealthWell Foundation

www.healthwellfoundation.org

Financial assistance for the underinsured. Provides aid for those with certain diseases who cannot afford their co-insurance, co-payments, health-care premiums, and deductibles for certain treatments.

Hill-Burton Free and Reduced Cost Health Care

www.hrsa.gov/hillburton/default.htm   (800) 638-0742

Facilities in the Hill-Burton program, which is administered by the federal government, can offer free or reduced-cost care to the uninsured.

The Leukemia & Lymphoma Society Co-pay Assistance Program

www.leukemia-lymphoma.org/all_page.adp?item_id=452658   (800) 955-4572

If you have a blood cancer and meet program requirements, the Leukemia & Lymphoma Society has a co-pay assistance program that will reimburse co-pays for doctor visits and prescriptions up to a certain amount. The society also reimburses travel and parking expenses; ask your hospital's social worker for a signed remittance form.

National Breast and Cervical Cancer Early Detection Program (NBCCEDP)

www.cdc.gov/cancer/NBCCEDP

This Centers for Disease Control and Prevention program provides access to critical breast and cervical cancer screening services to underserved women. Federal guidelines are generally at or below 250 percent of the federal poverty level, and eligible ages are eighteen to sixty-four for cervical screening and forty to sixty-four for breast screening. Some states extend their programs outside these parameters.

National Organization for Rare Disorders— Patient Assistance Programs

www.rarediseases.org/programs/medication
(203) 744-0100
Administers programs that provide assistance to patients with rare disorders (including some cancers) who are underinsured or uninsured and need help securing lifesaving or life-sustaining medications.

NCI Resources for Financial Assistance for Patients and Their Families

www.cancer.gov/cancertopics/factsheet/Support/
financial-resources
Searchable database of financial-assistance resources, available in English and Spanish.

Needy Meds

www.needymeds.org
Helps consumers fill in the individual pharmaceutical applications in search of free medications for their particular illness. You can see if your medication is available from this program at its Web site. Needy Meds also offers a database of free or low-cost clinics by state.

The Partnership for Prescription Assistance

www.pparx.org   (888) 477-2669
Mirrors what Needy Meds offers to consumers but allows you to search for multiple medications at once.

Patient Access Network Foundation

www.panfoundation.org
(866) 316-PANF (800-316-7263)
Provides assistance to patients through twenty-one disease-specific funds, including several cancers.

Rise Above It

www.raibenefit.org/
Offers financial assistance via grants to young adults, particularly those participating in clinical trials.

RX Assist

http://rxassist.org
A resource center with information about patient-assistance programs, primarily those administered by the drug companies themselves.

Travel Assistance

The Air Care Alliance

www.aircareall.org/   (888) 260-9707
Volunteer pilot organization that does charitable air transport.

Air Charity Network

www.aircharitynetwork.org   (877) 621-7177
National charitable aviation network.

Angel Flights

www.angelflight.com/   (918) 749-8992
Oklahoma-based volunteer pilot network offering free air transport to medical treatment, primarily in the heartland region.

Corporate Angel Network

www.corpangelnetwork.org   (866) 328-1313
Free air transport for cancer patients in empty seats on corporate jets.

National Patient Travel Center

www.patienttravel.org/index.html   (800) 296-1217
Travel resources for patients, including travel help line, charitable air travel, volunteer pilot organization, air ambulance coordination, and travel for escorts of patients.

Lodging Assistance

Hope Lodge

www.cancer.org/docroot/subsite/hopelodge/index.asp
(800) ACS-2345 (800-227-2345)
Hope Lodges, sponsored by the American Cancer Society, can be found near treatment centers in select locations. They offer free lodging in a nurturing environment and provide support services to patients traveling away from home to receive cancer treatment. The Web site also includes housing resources.

Joe's House

www.joeshouse.org   877-JOESHOU (877-563-7468)
Service that helps cancer patients find lodging near their treatment centers.

Miracle House

www.miraclehouse.org   (212) 989-7790
Temporary housing and support for patients receiving critical medical care in New York City.

National Association of Hospital Hospitality Houses

www.nahhh.org/

Provides services to hospitality houses and helps families find lodging and other support services near treatment facilities.

Disability and Work Information

Caring Connections

www.Caringinfo.org   (800) 658-8898

Multilingual line: (877) 658-8896

Get free downloadable advance directive forms; easy enough for a first grader.

Disability Secrets

www.disabilitysecrets.com

Site written by a former disability examiner, with tips, tricks, and information on Social Security Disability Insurance (SSDI) benefits that may not be found on the government's official Web site.

Landay, David S. *Be Prepared: The Complete Financial, Legal, and Practical Guide to Living with Cancer, HIV, and Other Life-Challenging Conditions.* New York: St. Martin's Press, 1998.

Larschan, Edward J., and Richard J. Larschan. *The Diagnosis Is Cancer: A Psychological and Legal Resource Handbook for Cancer Patients, Their Families, and Helping Professionals.* New York: Bull Publishing Company, 1986.

Social Security Administration

www.ssa.gov   (800) 772-1213

Apply for Social Security Disability Insurance (SSDI) online, check the status of and manage your disability application, answer your questions about disability, appeal your denied claim, check your eligibility for benefits using the online screening tool, and more. This site has a wealth of information; the amount of information, however, might be overwhelming.

Chapter 3—Treatment

Chemotherapy

Chemocare.com

www.chemocare.com

Who knew that figure-skating gold medalist Scott Hamilton would have such an extensive resource about chemotherapy? Offers incredibly comprehensive information about the drugs, the side effects, and managing them.

Chemotherapy.com

www.chemotherapy.com

Yes, this site is provided by a pharmaceutical company, but it's still chock-full of good, easily understandable information about chemotherapy: what it is, how it works, and potential side effects.

Dollinger, Malin, Ernest H. Rosenbaum, and Greg Cable. *Everyone's Guide to Cancer Therapy: How Cancer Is Diagnosed, Treated, and Managed Day to Day,* Revised Fifth Edition. Kansas City, Missouri: Andrews McMeel Publishing, 2008.

Radiation

Radiology Info

www.radiologyinfo.org

The public information Web site developed and funded by the American College of Radiology and the Radiological Society of North America. Information and details on how radiation is used in cancer treatment as well as in various diagnostic scans and tests.

Transplants

BMT InfoNet

www.bmtinfonet.org   (888) 597-7674

A service of the Blood & Marrow Transplant Information Network, providing transplant information, a transplant center directory, and patient-to-survivor matching program.

National Foundation for Transplants

www.transplants.org   (800) 489-3863

Allows transplant patients to receive tax-deductible donations through its foundation.

Clinical Trials

CenterWatch Clinical Trials Listing Service

www.centerwatch.com   (866) 219-3440

Source of information about clinical trials for patients and clinical trials industry professionals.

ClincialTrials.com

www.clinicaltrials.com

Information source for study participants detailing the ins and outs of clinical trials, including questions to ask your doctors, FAQs, podcasts, and a glossary of terms. In the "Knowledge Center" section, you can search for articles from a variety of sources.

ClinicalTrials.gov

http://clinicaltrials.gov

Search this federal government database, a service of the National Institutes for Health, for current trials specific to your disease.

LIVESTRONG SurvivorCare

www.livestrong.org

866-673-7205

Connect to a clinical trials matching service supported by Emerging Med.

NCI Clinical Trials Site

www.cancer.gov/clinicaltrials

(800) 4-CANCER (800-422-6237)

The National Cancer Institute's clinical trials site, which includes information on how to find trials, past research, and other resources for patients and researchers.

TrialCheck

www.cancertrialshelp.org

Clinical trials matching service provided by the Coalition of Cancer Cooperative Groups.

Chapter 4—Side Effects
Supportive Care

American Brain Tumor Association: Help with Side Effects—Radiation Therapy

www.abta.org/Treating_Brain_Tumors/
Help_with_Side_Effects_-_Radiation_Therapy/105

Information on living with the potential side effects of radiation therapy.

Chemocare.com

www.chemocare.com

A thorough resource about chemotherapy side effects and how to manage them.

Clegg, Ellen. *Chemo Brain: How Cancer Therapies Can Affect Your Mind.* Amherst, New York: Prometheus Books, 2009.

Gieringer, Dale, Ed Rosenthal, and Gregory T. Carter. *Marijuana Medical Handbook: Practical Guide to Therapeutic Uses of Marijuana.* Oakland, California: Quick Trading Co., 2008.

Rosenbaum, Ernest H., and Isadora Rosenbaum. *Everyone's Guide to Cancer Supportive Care: A Comprehensive Handbook for Patients and Their Families.* Kansas City, Missouri: Andrews McMeel Publishing, 2005.

Silverman, Dan, and Idelle Davidson. *Your Brain after Chemo: A Practical Guide to Lifting the Fog and Getting Back Your Focus.* Cambridge, Massachusetts: Da Capo Press, 2009.

Chapter 5—Staying Sane
Exercise

Hoffman, Lisa, with Alison Freeland. *The Healing Power of Movement: How to Benefit from Physical Activity During Your Cancer Treatment.* Cambridge, Massachusetts: Perseus Publishing. 2002.

Yoga Bear

www.yogabear.org

Nonprofit that promotes healing and wellness through yoga, specifically for those with cancer. Includes how-to videos, resources, forums, and financial assistance for survivors seeking free yoga classes in their area.

Food and Nutrition

Clegg, Holly, and Gerald Miletello. *Eating Well Through Cancer: Easy Recipes & Recommendations During & After Treatment.* Nashville, Tennessee: Favorite Recipes Press, 2006.

Ghosh, Kris, Linda Carson, and Elyse Cohen. *Betty Crocker's Living with Cancer Cookbook: Easy Recipes and Tips through Treatment and Beyond.* New York: Hungry Minds, 2002.

Sexuality and Intimacy

The American Association of Sexuality Educators, Counselors, and Therapists
www.aasect.org

American Cancer Society Sexuality for the Man with Cancer
www.cancer.org/docroot/MIT/MIT_7_1x_Sexuality
forMenandTheirPartners.asp

American Cancer Society Sexuality for the Woman with Cancer
www.cancer.org/docroot/MIT/MIT_7_1x_Sexuality
forWomenandTheirPartners.asp

Kroll, Ken, and Erica Klein Levy. *Enabling Romance: A Guide to Love, Sex, and Relationships for the Disabled (And the People Who Care About Them)*. Bethesda, Maryland: Woodbine House, 1995.

Laken, Virginia and Keith. *Making Love Again: Hope for Couples Facing Loss of Sexual Intimacy*. Sandwich, Massachusetts: Ant Hill Press, 2002.

The Leukemia & Lymphoma Society Fact Sheet on Sexuality and Intimacy
www.leukemia-lymphoma.org/attachments/National/
br_1208892732.pdf

National Cancer Institute: Sexuality and Reproductive Issues
www.cancer.gov/cancertopics/pdq/supportivecare/
sexuality
At this link, the NCI examines sexuality and reproductive issues as affected by cancer.

National LGBT Cancer Network
www.cancer-network.org/
Educating the LGBT community about cancer risks, training health-care providers on culturally competent care, and advocating for LGBT survivors.

Out with Cancer
www.outwithcancer.com
LGBT cancer information and support.

Sexual Health Network
www.sexualhealth.com
Dedicated to providing easy access to sexuality information, education, support, and other resources.

Schover, Leslie R. *Sexuality and Fertility after Cancer*. New York: John Wiley and Sons, 1997.

———, and Soren Buus Jensen. *Sexuality and Chronic Illness: A Comprehensive Approach*. New York: The Guilford Press, 1988.

Enhancement Aids and Information
You aren't going to get a bunch of porn pop-ups or e-mails from these groups (unless you want to!)
www.goodvibes.com; www.babeland.com; www.libida
.com; www.bettersex.com; www.pureromance.com
(Pure Romance has a survivorship section on its Web site: Click on "Programs.")

Fashion and Beauty
Gafni, Ramy. *Ramy Gafni's Beauty Therapy: The Ultimate Guide to Looking and Feeling Great While Living with Cancer*. New York: M. Evans & Company, 2005.

Ovitz, Lori M. *Facing the Mirror with Cancer: A Guide to Using Makeup to Make a Difference*. Chicago: Belle Press, 2004.

Complementary and Alternative Medicine
Alschuler, Lise N., and Karolyn A. Gazella. *Alternative Medicine Magazine's Definitive Guide to Cancer: An Integrated Approach to Prevention, Treatment, and Healing*. Berkeley, California: Celestial Arts, 2007.

American Cancer Society's Complete Guide to Complementary and Alternative Cancer Therapies, Second Edition. Atlanta: American Cancer Society, 2009.

Kris Carr: Crazy Sexy Cancer Tips and Crazy Sexy Wellness
www.crazysexylife.com
Kris Carr is a great voice for alternative approaches to fighting cancer, encouraging readers, for example, to be "Veggie Vixens." Learn more on her site.

M. D. Anderson Cancer Center Complementary/Integrative Medicine Education Resources
www.mdanderson.org/education-and-research/
resources-for-professionals/clinical-tools-and-
resources/cimer/index.html
Helps patients and physicians decide how best to integrate complementary and alternative medicine therapies into their care.

Memorial Sloan-Kettering Cancer Center: About Herbs, Botanicals, and Other Products

www.mskcc.org/mskcc/html/11570.cfm

This Web page's goal is to provide "objective information for oncologists and health-care professionals, including a clinical summary for each agent and details about constituents, adverse effects, interactions, and potential benefits or problems. Evaluations of alternative or unproved cancer therapies, as well as products for sexual dysfunction, are included."

National Center for Complementary and Alternative Medicine

http://nccam.nih.gov

Lots of information about various CAM approaches, from specifics about certain herbs to explanations about the benefits of acupuncture and probiotics.

Chapter 6—People
Communication Tools for Family and Friends

Babcock, Elise NeeDell. *When Life Becomes Precious: The Essential Guide for Patients, Loved Ones, and Friends of Those Facing Serious Illnesses.* New York: Bantam Books, 2002.

CarePages

www.carepages.org

A resource center with tips for you and your loved ones on how to communicate during a health crisis (major!!), articles and inspirational stories, discussion forums, and helpful blogs written by experts. CarePages also has a gift shop powered by Amazon.com that offers gift suggestions listed by recipient or situation.

CaringBridge

www.caringbridge.org

Free personal Web pages for people fighting illness. Keep a personal online journal, post photos, and allow friends and family members to sign your guestbook. CaringBridge also offers a service that turns your online journal into a bound book for a small fee.

Grinyer, Anne. *Cancer in Young Adults: Through Parents' Eyes.* Buckingham, U.K.: Open University Press, 2002.

Hope, Lori. *Help Me Live: 20 Things People with Cancer Want You to Know.* Berkeley, California: Celestial Arts, 2005.

Lotsa Helping Hands

www.lotsahelpinghands.org

Lotsa Helping Hands is a free coordination site for friends and family of those in need. Set up a calendar and list appointments, errands, or chores, and loved ones sign up for tasks they are able to help with at their convenience.

My LifeLine

www.mylifeline.org

Set up a page where family and friends can leave messages and donate money to offset the costs of treatment. Set up a calendar, search a resources directory and glossary of medical terms, consolidate all your e-mail and pick it up here, and enjoy inspirational quotes and humor to help get you through tough days.

Peterson, Cathy. *Call Me If You Need Anything . . . and Other Things Not to Say: A Guide to Helping Others through Tragedy and Grief.* St. Louis, Missouri: Chalice Press, 2005.

Connecting with Other Young Adults
Gilda's Club

www.gildasclub.org

Network of clubhouses that provide social support for cancer patients and survivors of all ages around the world. Many Gilda's Clubs offer networking groups for young adults.

Imerman Angels (877) 274-5529

www.imermanangels.org

Imerman Angels matches cancer patients with survivors of their same age, gender, and cancer type. We couldn't create a better FAN if we tried.

I'm Too Young for This!

http://i2y.com/

Web portal of many sites for young adults with cancer. Home of the *Stupid Cancer* radio show.

Planet Cancer

www.planetcancer.org (512) 236-8820

Peer support and advocacy resources under the umbrella of **LIVESTRONG,** including the world's largest social network for young adults with cancer.

Young Survival Coalition

www.youngsurvival.org/ (877) YSC-1011
(877-972-1011)

Organization dedicated to young breast cancer survivors.

Retreats and Camps for Young Adults

Camp Mak-A-Dream

http://campdream.org (406) 549-5987

Weeklong programs for young adults with cancer, siblings, and young adult survivor advocate training.

First Descents

www.firstdescents.org (970) 926-2444

Kayaking and outdoor adventure retreats for young adults ages eighteen to thirty-nine.

Minnie Pearl Cancer Foundation Young Adult Cancer Survivor Retreat

http://minniepearl.org/programs (615) 467-1936

Nashville-based retreats for young adults with cancer.

Next Step

www.nextstepnet.org (617) 864-2921

Weekend programs for young adults with cancer, young couples, and care-dependent survivors with their caregivers.

Planet Cancer Retreats

www.planetcancer.org
(512) 226-8820

The original. Weekend programs for young adults with cancer and young couples facing cancer together.

For Families with Kids

Harpham, Wendy Schlessel. *When a Parent Has Cancer: A Guide to Caring for Your Children*. New York: HarperCollins, 1997.

Kids Konnected

www.kidskonnected.org

This nonprofit aims to help children whose parents have cancer. Information for children, teens, parents, and professionals. The Web site has an online chat room for kids, a therapist whom parents can e-mail, and support group locations. Kids Konnected also provides a 24/7 hotline for kids manned by trained "youth leaders" ages fourteen to eighteen, who answer questions or just talk to callers. The organization also hosts summer camps for kids of all ages.

SuperSibs

www.supersibs.org
(866) 444-SIBS (866-444-7427)

Organization for brothers and sisters (adolescent or younger) of children or adolescents with cancer. Includes scholarship programs, resources for parents, and more.

For Young Spouses

Young Cancer Spouses

www.youngcancerspouses.com

Resources for spouses of young adults with cancer.

Chapter 7—What Now?

Work Issues

Cancer and Careers

www.cancerandcareers.org

An invaluable resource on cancer in the workplace, including tips for interviewing, what your employer can and can't do, fashion and beauty tips, and career coaches to help you through work-related transitions.

Life after Cancer

Carr, Kris. *Crazy Sexy Cancer Survivor: More Rebellion and Fire for Your Healing Journey*. Guilford, Connecticut: Skirt, 2008.

Dorfman, Elena, and Heidi Schultz Adams. *Here and Now: Inspiring Stories of Cancer Survivors*. New York: Marlowe & Company, 2002.

Feuerstein, Michael, and Patricia Findley. *The Cancer Survivor's Guide: The Essential Handbook to Life after Cancer*. New York: Marlowe & Company, 2006.

Grinyer, Anne. *Life after Cancer in Adolescence and Young Adulthood: The Experience of Survivorship*. New York: Routledge, 2009.

Rosenbaum, Ernest H., David Spiegel, Patricia Fobair, Holly Gautier, with Louise Maffitt. *Everyone's Guide to Cancer Survivorship: A Road Map for Better Health*. Kansas City, Missouri: Andrews McMeel Publishing, 2007.

Scholarships and Grants for Young Adults

The Brenda Mehling Cancer Fund
www.bmcf.net
Offers scholarships, support for living expenses, and financial assistance to adolescents and young adults undergoing treatment.

Cancer for College
www.cancerforcollege.org
(760) 599-5096

Cancer Survivors' Fund
www.cancersurvivorsfund.org
(281) 437-7142
Provides scholarships and financial aid for prosthetic limbs to young adult survivors.

FinAid: Financial Aid for Students with Disabilities
www.finaid.org/otheraid/disabled.phtml
(724) 538-4500

The Nicki Leach Foundation
www.nickileach.org
(904) 280-8916
Provides assistance and funding for special activities to high school and college-age survivors.

SAMFund
www.thesamfund.org
(866) 439-9365
The Surviving and Moving Forward Fund provides diverse and generous grants to help young adult cancer survivors meet their needs after treatment.

The Ulman Cancer Fund for Young Adults
www.ulmanfund.org
(888) 393-FUND (888-393-3863)
The Ulman Cancer Fund, founded by LIVE**STRONG** CEO Doug Ulman, offers scholarships to young adult survivors and visionary grants for related programs, in addition to its support groups and networks.

Working Against Cancer
www.workingagainstcancer.org
Provides scholarships for college and vocational training to young adult survivors whose past cancer treatment has interfered with education and work training.

Resources on Death and Dying

Beresford, Larry. *The Hospice Handbook: A Complete Guide.* New York: Little, Brown and Company, 1993.

Brody, Jane. *Jane Brody's Guide to the Great Beyond: A Practical Primer to Help You and Your Loved Ones Prepare Medically, Legally, and Emotionally for the End of Life.* New York: Random House, 2009.

Byock, Ira. *Dying Well: Peace and Possibilities at the End of Life.* New York: Riverhead Books, 1997.

Fleet, Carole Brody, with Syd Harriet. *Widows Wear Stilettos: A Practical and Emotional Guide for the Young Widow.* Far Hills, New Jersey: New Horizon Press, 2009.

Growth House
www.growthhouse.org/
Resources on death and dying, hospice, palliative care, and pain management.

Hospice Foundation of America
www.hospicefoundation.org
(800) 854-3402
Information about hospice and palliative care, choosing a hospice, and dispelling myths about hospice.

Kubler-Ross, Elisabeth. *On Death and Dying.* New York: Scribner Classics, 1997.

Kuhl, David. *What Dying People Want: Practical Wisdom for the End of Life.* New York: Public Affairs, 2002.

Lief, Judith L. *Making Friends with Death: A Buddhist Guide to Encountering Mortality.* Boston: Shambhala Publications, 2001.

Nuland, Sherwin B. *How We Die: Reflections on Life's Final Chapter.* New York: Alfred A. Knopf, 1994.

Young, Gary and Kathy. *Loss and Found: How We Survived the Loss of a Young Spouse.* Calabasas, California: Calabash Press, 2001.

adjuvant chemotherapy: Chemo after surgery to remove a tumor. Its purpose is to make sure the cancer remains gone.

advance directive: Documents to provide guidance for medical and health-care decisions in the event you become mentally incompetent to make such decisions or unable to communicate such decisions. (See "living will" and "medical power of attorney.")

alternative medicine: Practices used in place of conventional medicine.

basal body temperature (BBT): The body's temperature when measured immediately after you wake up, so as not to be altered by any activity.

cannula: A small tube used for insertion into a body cavity.

catheter: A thin plastic tube. When a catheter is placed in a vein, it provides a path for drugs, nutrients, or blood products to enter the body. When a catheter is placed in a body cavity, it provides a path to drain fluid from the body.

CHOP chemotherapy: A chemo combination of: C (cyclophosphamide); H (hydroxydoxorubicin, aka Adriamycin, aka the "Red Devil"); O (Oncovin, trade name for vincristine); and P (prednisone, a steroid and, some would argue, the worst part). It's typically used to treats non-Hodgkin's lymphoma.

clinical trial: A scientifically controlled study of the safety and effectiveness of a therapeutic agent (like a drug or vaccine) using consenting patients.

complementary medicine: A group of disciplines employed along with conventional medicine, such as using acupuncture to help control nausea from chemotherapy.

CT scan: Computed tomography scan. An imaging method that uses X-rays to create cross-sectional pictures of the body.

grade: Describes the aggressiveness of cancer cells (how fast they spread) using numerals I to IV. Grade I (low-grade) is the least belligerent; IV (high-grade) is the most.

G-tube (gastronomy tube): A gastric feeding tube that connects to the stomach via a small incision in the abdomen.

Hodgkin's disease: Also Hodgkin's lymphoma. Cancer of the lymphatic system, and one of the most common cancers in young adults. Specifically, Hodgkin's disease is characterized by maverick, infection-fighting B cells that, instead of dying (like normal cells), create more malformed cancerous cells.

integrative (or integrated) medicine: Combines treatments from conventional medicine and complementary and alternative medicine. The approach is a holistic one that involves the patient's mind, body, and spirit.

intubation: The process of putting a tube into a hollow organ or passageway, often into the airway.

IV: Stands for "intravenous," which means the administration of something—meds, nutrients, chemo, platelets, whatever—directly into a vein, sometimes from a syringe, sometimes as a fluid drip.

living will: A document that specifies what types of medical treatment you desire, for use if you become mentally incompetent or unable to communicate.

medical power of attorney: A document that designates the person to make medical decisions on your behalf.

metastasis: The spread of cancer from the original site of disease to another part of the body.

MUGA (multiple gated acquisition) scan: A test to monitor the health of your heart. Adriamycin, a common chemotherapy drug, can be pretty tough on your heart; this procedure allows physicians to monitor a heart's health during treatment. The test itself involves an injection of (minimally!) radioactive red blood cells into the patient—these cells allow an image of the beating heart to be displayed on a monitor.

nasopharyngeal carcinoma (NPC): The most common tumor that affects the nasopharynx, which, besides sounding like a Dr. Seuss character, is a cavity triangulated by the base of your skull, the top of your soft palate, and the back of your nose.

neuropathy: When a peripheral nerve works poorly, is damaged, etc. Your limbs might feel weak or numb if you suffer from neuropathy.

neutropenia: When you have a low neutrophil count. (Neutrophils are the most important type of infection-fighting white blood cell.) If your absolute neutrophil count (ANC) is below 1,000, you are probably neutropenic, and are particularly susceptible to infections.

palliative care: A treatment that may relieve symptoms without curing the disease.

pathology report: A lab's analysis of tissue, blood, or other substances from your body. Relevant here is that the report contains your diagnosis, which the pathologist on your medical team has arrived at by checking out the tumor sample secured via biopsy or surgery.

PET scan: Stands for "positron emission tomography." An imaging test that uses a radioactive substance (known as a "tracer") to look for disease in the body.

PDQ (Physician's Data Query): A cancer database compiled by the National Cancer Institute. It includes basic information, treatment summaries (both patient and physician versions), and a registry of thousands of clinical trials from around the world.

platelet: An element in the blood that assists in clotting.

port-a-cath: A small medical appliance installed beneath the skin and used to provide long-term IV access to administer TPN, blood products, drugs, and chemotherapy.

PubMed: An online service of the U.S. National Library of Medicine. It provides links to millions of journal articles and other biomedical resources.

R-CHOP chemotherapy: CHOP chemo with the addition of the drug rituximab.

red blood cells: The most common type of blood cell and the means of delivering oxygen to the body's tissues.

seminoma: One of the two primary types of testicular cancer (the other is, appropriately, nonseminoma). Seminomas are less common and don't grow as quickly as nonseminomas; they also are more susceptible to being zapped by radiation.

stage: Describes how far cancer has spread. Overall groupings describe a cancer's stage with numerals I to IV: I indicates a localized tumor, and IV indicates metastatic cancer, or cancer that has spread.

subcutaneous: Beneath or under all the layers of the skin.

survivorship care plan: A plan put together following treatment that outlines the long-term side effects you may experience, as well as what type of screening tests you should get and how often to get them.

total parenteral nutrition (TPN): Nutritional formulas that you can receive through your catheter when you can't get food down. They provide your body with nutrients such as salts, glucose, amino acids, lipids, and vitamins.

tumor block: A sample of tumorous tissue preserved during a clinical trial for further study.

tumor markers: Substances found in your blood, urine, or tissue (it can be the tumor tissue, but it might be other tissue) that help diagnose your cancer and stage; when you're in treatment, tumor markers help gauge your response to treatment.

white blood cells: Cells of the immune system that defend the body against infectious disease and foreign materials.

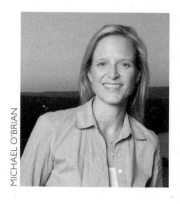

MICHAEL O'BRIAN

Heidi Schultz Adams is the founder and executive director of Planet Cancer, a community of advocacy and support for young adults with cancer, which she launched in 2001 after her own treatment at twenty-six for a rare type of bone cancer called Ewing's sarcoma. She founded Planet Cancer in response to her personal experience of the void in information and support services for younger adults under forty.

She is a founding member and the advocacy chair of the Lance Armstrong Foundation's LIVE**STRONG** Young Adult Alliance, a national coalition of more than one hundred organizations dedicated to improving survival rates and quality of life for young adults with cancer. In 2005, she received the prestigious LIVE**STRONG** Award, and in 2006 she was named a Swiffer Amazing Woman of the Year. In 2007 she was named one of four national Health Heroes by *WebMD* magazine and, in 2009 she was awarded the Lane Adams Quality of Life Award by the national American Cancer Society, given "to recognize and reward individuals who innovatively and consistently provide excellent and compassionate skilled care, counsel, and/or service to persons with cancer and their families."

A writer by profession, Heidi is also a contributor and editorial advisor to *CURE* magazine and is the coauthor of *Here and Now: Inspiring Stories of Cancer Survivors*, published in 2001 by Avalon and featured in *O: The Oprah Magazine*. She lives in Austin, Texas.

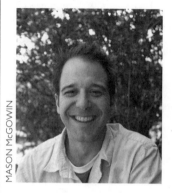

MASON McGOWIN

Christopher Schultz's fiction and nonfiction have appeared in *Esquire*, the *New York Times*, *Men's Journal*, *ESPN The Magazine*, *Spin*, *Shenandoah*, and other publications. He is coauthor of *The Yo Momma Vocabulary Builder*, a book featured in the *New York Times*, *Newsweek*, and on *ABC News* that teaches SAT words by using "Yo momma" jokes.

Christopher is the founder of Start Here Project Development, which helps businesses, nonprofits, and universities bring their ideas to reality through strategy and fund-raising, and strengthens these entities' communications. He spent much of 2010 as writer-in-residence at the Fairhope Center for the Writing Arts in Fairhope, Alabama, where he worked on a novel.